Mediumship
Within

Mediumship Within

Chris Ratter

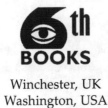

6th
BOOKS

Winchester, UK
Washington, USA

First published by Sixth Books, 2016
Sixth Books is an imprint of John Hunt Publishing Ltd., Laurel House, Station Approach,
Alresford, Hants, SO24 9JH, UK
office1@jhpbooks.net
www.johnhuntpublishing.com
www.6th-books.com

For distributor details and how to order please visit the 'Ordering' section on our website.

ISBN: 978 1 78535 334 5
Library of Congress Control Number: 2015954377

A CIP catalogue record for this book is available from the British Library.

Design: Stuart Davies

Printed and bound by CPI Group (UK) Ltd, Croydon, CR0 4YY, UK

We operate a distinctive and ethical publishing philosophy in all
areas of our business, from our global network of authors to
production and worldwide distribution.

CONTENTS

Acknowledgements

Many thanks to my beautiful wife Gail, my gorgeous daughter Natalie and my strapping son Connor. Without their encouragement I would probably not have completed this part of my journey.

To my spiritual guides Harry Edwards, Kao Chu and Grey Horse, for their direction in instigating this book and for their trust and belief in me.

To Pauline and John Hamley, Pauline Garden and Eric Brock for all their hard work, professionalism and patience in bringing this book to fruition.

Finally a special thanks to everyone mentioned in this book, for allowing me to use their names and experiences. They have helped me along my spiritual path.

Preface

I never thought that I would be working as a spiritual healer, let alone as a Psychic Surgeon, carrying out the work that I do today on behalf of the Divine Spirit and the workers from the Spirit World. This part of my life has been a wonderful awakening to me and I feel so blessed that I can share my experiences with you. This book is about my development within the healing side of mediumship. My purpose in writing it is to provide help and guidance to those who are thinking about following the path into spiritual healing, trance and trance healing mediumship.

Throughout my journey I have been faced with many questions and doubts. However, over time, wonderful people have come forward from the Spirit side of life, in love and trust, to work with me. They have provided me with information that has helped to develop my understanding of what has been taking place throughout my spiritual journey into this, the unseen side of life, which seems so far removed to many people.

At the start of my journey I never really knew of the existence of the Spirit World. If it had not been for the evidence that was brought through by spirit guides and healers, when they felt I was ready to receive it, I would be unaware of it still. Now, when I look back over my life and remember certain things that took place as I was growing up, I can understand their significance. However, at the time, since there was no one to explain them to me, just like any other child growing up, I would tend to dismiss what I had been shown or was aware of concerning the Spirit World.

A Dawning Awareness of Spirit

Childhood Experiences

My earliest memory of spirit people, or shadow people as some like to call them, was when I was a very young child. My parents, two sisters and I lived in a council flat in an area of Edinburgh called Wardieburn. I remember waking up one night and seeing people walking down the hall beyond the open bedroom door, heading in the direction of the bathroom. This happened on several occasions as I lay awake and watched. To be honest, I was terrified. Eventually I mustered the courage to wake one of my sisters and together we went to have a look in the bathroom. There was no one there. I would see these shadow people walk down the hall almost every night.

The next experience that I can recall from memory was when I was staying at my grandparents' house. I would stay with them almost every weekend and I would sleep in their bedroom on bunk beds at the side of their double bed. I remember waking my granny up most of the nights that I stayed there because there were people (shadow people) in the room. This always resulted in her comforting me. 'They won't hurt you,' she would say. 'In you come to my bed.' I always found this to be very reassuring. I have really enjoyable memories of the visits to my grandparents.

I spent quite a lot of time by myself wandering around the grounds of the castle that my grandfather looked after and never really felt alone. Often I would be aware of speaking to myself in my own mind. I was constantly asking questions, and sometimes I would hear an answer. To keep myself amused when I was wandering around on my own I used to play a game in my mind. Now I can understand what it was that I was doing but at the time it was a just a game to me to see how far I could shift my consciousness to the side. Sometimes I was able to shift my consciousness (which felt like I had entered into another world or

2

dimension) to such a degree that I would feel as if I was going to faint.

'A strange game for a child to play,' I can hear you say. Nevertheless, it was a game that I liked to play when I was on my own. I did not know that even back then my spirit friends were conducting experiments with me involving the altered states of trance. It was not until later on in my life, when I had some experience of trance mediumship, that I was able to begin to understand what had been happening all those years before.

Another game that I used to play involved heat through my hands. I would ask one of my sisters to lay her arms on the floor and I would put my hand over her arm or hand. I would then request that the part of their body under my hand to heat up. 'Heat up, heat up, heat up,' I would say, and then, 'go cold, go cold.' Afterwards, I would return to, 'Heat up, heat up.' My sisters were always up for this, but after a while it would start to 'freak them out' and the game would stop. I now know that this was the Spirit World getting me to experiment with the use of using spiritual healing energy.

Children are innocent when it comes to all things spiritual. When a child has an imaginary friend it may be imaginary to us, but it will seem very real to them. Children do not dismiss the Spirit World as easily as we do; they are openly receptive to whatever they see, feel and become aware of. Their minds have not been conditioned like those of adults. Children's minds and thoughts are pure and uncorrupted. They are willing to accept anything and everything, seen and unseen, in our physical world. It is not uncommon for a child to tell their parents that they have spoken to loved ones (grandparents) who have visited them during the night or through the day. Often these loved ones have passed into the Spirit World before the child was born. Nonetheless the child is able to pick them out from a photograph.

Adults and parents should encourage their children to have

an open mind concerning the Spirit World. They should recognize that it is acceptable for children to have imaginary friends. I have never heard of an imaginary friend causing a problem for a child. The problem usually arises due to the parent or guardian failing to understand, or to accept, what is happening. The people from the Spirit World are never going to harm anyone. They are love, nothing less, and they only want to bring that love to those of us on the material plane, together with the understanding that we are all connected through the love of Divine Spirit.

Like many people who were visited by the spirit people at an early age, these weird but wonderful experiences started to leave me as grew older. Eventually they ceased altogether. This is a common occurrence for people who are aware of Spirit when they are very young. I suppose that one of the reasons for this happening is that not all children are aware of the Spirit World, and when we go to school children are all too willing to ridicule any child who is a little different. The Spirit World is all about protecting and supporting. It is not about hurting.

I was lucky to have grandparents who were supportive and who had an understanding of the unseen world of Spirit. The next time a parent scolds a child for speaking to an 'imaginary friend', I ask that they consider that perhaps the imaginary friend is not so imaginary after all. I was very privileged to be able to spend lots of time with my grandparents when I was young. My grandfather came to live with us when my granny passed over to the Spirit World. He was responsible for introducing me to Spiritualist churches at a young age. These churches always seemed familiar to me and I felt very comfortable in the surroundings. I loved to watch the medium from the platform speaking to the shadow people and talking about people's loved ones who were no longer of this world. I have no doubt that my granddad was well aware that there was something different about me, and that this is why he encouraged me to attend these spiritualist organizations (in order that I would know where to turn to when the time was right).

Reintroduction to the World of Spirit

I was thirty-eight years of age when the Spirit World decided that it was time for them to reintroduce themselves into my life. One evening, when I was lying in my bed watching television, I started to see shadow people out of the corner of my eye. This began as movement that would catch my attention, but I was never able to lock onto what I was seeing or feeling.

Another evening, when I was going to sleep, as I closed my eyes a bright light seemed to come on in the room. I remember opening my eyes, expecting to see one of my children standing by the door, but to my surprise the only thing I saw was a pitch black room. 'Strange,' I thought to myself, and closed my eyes again. A few minutes later the bright white light returned. Again I opened my eyes to find the room in total darkness. This time I remember exclaiming, 'What the hell is going on?' as I put my head back onto the pillow to tried to get back to sleep. Once again the light was there. This time I just tried to ignore it and eventually managed to get to sleep. When I woke in the morning I remember thinking to myself, 'What was all that all about?'

That evening I went back to work, driving my hackney cab on the nightshift. I got home about five o'clock in the morning. As I entered my home I could smell pipe smoke. This smell reminded me of my grandfather, who had been a pipe smoker all the time that I had known him. When I then turned to switch off the house alarm system I saw a young boy standing at the top of the staircase. At first I thought it was my son who was about the same size and build as the child who was standing at the top of the stairs. However, this was not the case. The apparition disappeared. I attributed what I had witnessed to feeling tired after my nightshift, proceeded to the kitchen and made myself a cup of tea. Roughly an hour later I retired to my bedroom to get some sleep.

A Fright in the Night

The bedroom was in total darkness. My wife, Gail, was asleep. Not wishing to disturb her I did not put the light on. I climbed into bed, closed my eyes and snuggled into the pillow. A few minutes later the bright, white light appeared once again. Eyes open, light gone. Eyes closed, light on. I could not understand what was happening to me. I was starting to think that perhaps I was going mad. Due to the light show, I was getting very little sleep.

A few weeks passed with these strange bright lights appearing in my eyes every night. Hoping that these events would cease as suddenly as they had started, and that things would return to normal, I told no one about them. Instead they got worse. The bedroom felt as though a freezer door was open at my side of the bed. I knew that there was something nearby that was the cause of the light show, and of the cold air that was blowing onto me, but I was trying to ignore it. The lights would start to shine whenever I closed my eyes. I was exhausted. Then one evening I heard voices in the room. My first thought was that it was Gail talking in her sleep, but she was sound asleep.

With all these things happening around me I was trying to keep a grip on reality, but with the lack of sleep this was becoming difficult. I think I managed to get a few hours of sleep that night, but not enough to function properly. I was becoming really concerned about everything that was happening and was considering going to see my doctor concerning the problem.

'I'm speaking to you!'

That evening, when I went to bed everything was just the same. Lights appeared in my eyes and an ice-cold breeze blew at the side of my bed. I tried to ignore everything and go to sleep, but a few hours later I heard voices once again in the room. 'Wake up! Wake up! I'm speaking to you,' I heard loudly. This startled me. I sat up, looked around the room and saw people standing at the bottom of my bed, not shadow people like before, but real spirit people standing watching Gail and me lying in bed. I sat as if frozen in time, looking at these people in my bedroom standing at the bottom of my bed. Then one of the figures came forward towards me at the side of the bed, turned to their left and proceeded to walk through the bedroom door.

That was enough for me. Now I was petrified and proceeded to scramble to Gail's side of the bed for protection. Gail woke up and angrily asked what was going on. I thought to myself, 'I'm just going to tell her everything that's been going on, and if I'm nuts then I'm nuts.' Gail listened as I told her about everything that had been happening during the last few months. She cuddled into me and said that everything would be all right. 'Easy for you to say that, when nothing is happening to you,' I thought.

The following evening we spoke at length about my experiences before retiring to bed. I felt better after discussing my problem with Gail. If she thought I was going mad then, bless her, she kept it to herself. That night was just the same. I tried to stay awake as long as possible to avoid a recurrence of the phenomena, but by now I was exhausted. Eventually I fell asleep. Once again, I heard a voice shouting loudly, 'I'm speaking to you! I'm speaking to you!' This startled me. I opened my eyes, but this time it felt as if I was being strangled. I panicked and flung myself in the general direction of Gail, startling her out of her sleep. 'What the hell is going on?' she demanded. After explaining to her what had happened, we settled back into bed and fell asleep. Once again the voice was back, together with the feeling of being strangled.

To be truthful, with all the events that had been happening over the last few months, I was really scared. A member of my family had been diagnosed with schizophrenia a few months before all this had started happening to me, and I was concerned that the condition may be hereditary. The following day, when

Gail arrived home from her work, I told her that I wanted to go to a spiritualist church. This was something that we had never talked about in all the years we had been together. We checked the web and found a church that had a service that evening. At the time I had no idea that I was embarking upon a journey that would change the rest of my life.

Help is at Hand

We went to the church service, not knowing what to expect. We sat in the audience and I received messages from the medium on the platform about not missing the bus, confirmation that my grandparents were around, and nonsense about healing hands. To be honest it all sounded a bit sketchy to me. After the service we went for a coffee and a biscuit in the cafe inside the church premises. I managed to speak to a lady who explained to us that although she was not a medium, she was a committee member of the church. She listened intently to what I had to say regarding these strange events that had been going on in my life over the last few months, and tried her best to give me an explanation for what was happening around about me. However, we came away with many unanswered questions.

The following evening Gail and I went to a service at another spiritualist church to seek a better explanation concerning the things that had been happening around me. This service was held inside a town hall, not a church. We paid an entrance fee and sat on two seats at the back of the congregation. The female medium started the service with a prayer, and we watched as she paced up and down in front of the seating arrangements giving out messages of existence of life after death from their loved ones in the Spirit World to members of the audience who seemed to be very happy with the information they were receiving from her.

When the lady had finished passing messages to the audience, and she had brought the proceedings of the evening to a close, I went to speak to her. She kindly took the time to listen to what I had to say. 'You're not mad,' she told me, 'you do know that. There're too many spirit people around you for them just to be family members.' She went on to say that the mad ones are the people who come and tell her that they are hearing voices behind the curtains, couches, in the walls and under the floor boards.

'What is happening to you is that you have become aware of Spirit, and they have become aware of you,' she explained. 'Although you do not realize it, you are emitting a beacon of white light. It is invisible to the human eye, but to those in the Spirit World it's a beacon that lets them know you can communicate with them, and this is what's happening to you. They are drawn to the light, and you're becoming aware of them as they draw close to you.'

'What do I do to stop it?' I asked. 'Tell them to F**k off!' was her reply. I was dumbfounded at this answer from her. I had just watched this lady talking about the Divine Spirit and the love that comes from the Spirit World with an audience of about forty people listening, and hanging on to every word she had been saying to them. However, it was a firm answer. I needed firm answers concerning everything that I had been experiencing, and this firm approach made sense to me.

'I will show you how to protect yourself through a white light exercise,' she said. 'It may take up to a week for you to get things under control, but eventually it will stop them from coming forward and disturbing your sleep pattern.' I thanked the lady for her honesty. This conversation with her had settled my mind. What a relief to hear someone tell me I was not mad, and give me an explanation for the strange events that had started in my life!

That evening I started the exercise involving light protection, as instructed. As she had predicted, just over a week later everything was under control. Although the strange events of the previous few months had scared me at first, now that I had a very limited understanding of what had taken place I decided to investigate further. Everything that had taken place with me had stirred my interest. A couple of weeks later I had joined the lady's mental mediumship development circle.

The Gift of Mediumship

A Calling to Serve

Mediumship, in all its many forms, is a calling to serve Divine Spirit, the Universal Energy or whatever you wish to call it, and must not be taken lightly. The gift of mediumship can only manifest itself when the time is right, both for you and for Spirit. Spirit people will only come into your life when the time is right for your gift to unfold, and for your spiritual journey to begin. We have the right to accept them into our lives or to shut them out. Everyone has this freedom of choice, even those people from the spirit side of life.

When you first start to look into the beautiful gift of mediumship it is advisable to keep an open mind concerning all things, seen and unseen. Try not to be judgmental concerning whatever you may experience, sense or feel. I have no doubt in saying to you that many weird and wonderful things will be shown to you from the World of Spirit. At first you will not understand them, but as your awareness and curiosity start to expand, you will begin to look more deeply into these strange, but wonderful, inexplicable experiences that are happening around you.

I have no hesitation in telling you that the Spirit World does exist. It is far closer to our world than we can possibly comprehend. Those who dwell in the Spirit World no longer have, or require, the use of a physical body. However, at one time they did have a physical body when they were living their lives here in the material world, before they returned home to the World of Spirit that we all come from. Yes, we all return home to the Spirit World after we have had our period of existence on this, the material world. Those who have gone through the transition of death, as we know it, have not ceased to exist. They have merely returned home to the Spirit World in the form of energy-based life forms.

The spirit or soul of each one of us, is contained within our physical body and is the true essence of who we really are. The physical body is only a vessel, a shell that allows us to experience a spiritual journey of awakening in this physical world in which we live. The purpose of our existence on this material world is to undergo life experiences in order to gain knowledge so that we can progress our spiritual growth.

Spiritual growth comes in many forms. At some time in our lives we all have to experience the loss of a family member, a loved one or a friend. These people may have been taken from us quickly, tragically, or they may had suffered with an illness that caused them to slowly wither away before us, over a long period of time. All of the emotions that we experience at this time are part of the healing process, and contribute to our spiritual development.

When a child is born into this world it brings forward a whole new set of emotions as family and friends rejoice at the birth of a new family member. You must remember that grief, stress, depression, strife, loneliness, fear, pain, happiness, love, joy, compassion, to name but a few, are feelings and emotions that we will all experience during our time in this world. They are necessary parts of the life experience, and all contribute to our spiritual growth.

Communication with Our Spirit Friends

One of the problems that spirit people have in making us aware of their presence, and in trying to communicate with us, is that in our daily lives we rely upon the five senses, of sight, hearing, touch, smell and taste to interact with our environment. We are used to living in a world in which everything appears to be 'black and white' for us. If we can sense it then it exists. Our minds are conditioned to ignore anything we cannot detect with our senses. When the Spirit World tries to introduce color into our lives, this can have a detrimental effect upon some people. For some it can start the mind spiraling off on a different train of thought. For others, the blinkers are on and they just ignore it.

We live in a world full of physical matter, energies and vibrations. These are all around us and everything seems solid to us. We go about our daily lives in a robotic state of consciousness, where we do the same things over and over again. We walk around feeling the firmness of the ground under our feet, the warmth of the sun as it heats up our bodies and the wind blowing through our hair on a breezy day. We have become accustomed to these things and, since they feel very familiar to us, we take them for granted.

Unfortunately, with the pace of modern living, we never really take the time to step back and to appreciate how beautiful our world truly is. Over time our minds have been programmed to carry out our daily duties without question. We have conditioned our minds not to look beyond the veil that separates our world from the World of Spirit. We easily dismiss the shadow figure of a person that we have seen out of the corner of our eye, and fail to acknowledge hearing our name being whispered in our ear when we are alone. Through time we have learned to dismiss these things and to put them all down to having a vivid imagination. That is easier than it is for us to accept those things that we cannot explain.

From the earliest times, some degree of communication with ascended life forms has been recognized and recorded. Why should it be any different today? The Spirit World hasn't disappeared. It is still there. The people who dwell in the Realm of Spirit have not stopped trying to communicate with us. In our busy lives we have become unreceptive to these messages, visions and inexplicable things that they send. Our loved ones, guides and protectors are constantly trying to communicate with us in any way that they can.

When they start to make their presence known, you may

begin to experience sensations such as ice-cold spots in certain areas of your home. You may also become aware of the smell of smoke or perfume. For some (as in my case) it may involve all of the above, together with the additional bonus of being able to see spirit people and to hear their voices.

We fail to appreciate the great effort that it takes those in the Spirit World to manifest these phenomena to the extent that we are able to experience them. To achieve these effects, considerable amounts of energy must be transferred from their world into ours, where these spirit workers must then manipulate it.

If you accept, and allow spirit people to come into your life, it will become your greatest journey of awakening. The energy that they bring will touch your heart. It will be filled with so much love and compassion for humankind that this will emanate from you like a beacon of white light, and will touch upon everyone that you meet on your journey.

The understanding that they will bring to you will help to free your mind, and will enable you to understand that all things are possible. It takes time to develop to become a working medium. It will not be an easy journey. We all have psychic abilities to a degree (to be able to feel and access information contained within other peoples' energy etc.). However, it takes time to be able to open a channel to the Spirit World in a controlled manner, in order to relay relevant information from Spirit with confidence.

Spirit Guides

I have no doubt in saying that your spirit guides have been with you for a long time, perhaps without your knowledge. They will know you very well, even if you are unaware of them. When you get to know them you may find that, unknown to you, you have been influenced by their presence for quite some time.

Many mediums constantly refer to the guides who work with them from the spirit side of life by name. During the course of my development I remember wondering why it was that these people all seemed to have guides with famous names like Sitting Bull, Red Cloud, and Merlin. Why can't a guide just be a normal person called Bob, George or something simple like that?

I think that people like to associate themselves with prominent figures from the past in order to make them, and their mediumship seem to be more important to other people and, in some cases, to themselves. It is not the guide's name that matters. In mediumship, what is important is the quality of the work that they can achieve through you. They may never give you their name, but does that really matter? I think not!

The spirit people who support us in the development and delivery of our mediumship come from diverse backgrounds. Not all will have lived previously on the Earth plane. However, those that have will be representative of all walks of life. Whatever their background these people bring experience and wisdom to assist and support us in our mediumship.

When we actively seek the name of one of our guides it is easy for us to make mistakes. The names that they were known by when they were on the Earth plane are unimportant to people in the Spirit World. We are only human and can sometimes get confused about what we are feeling and seeing. For example, if we are working with a spirit guide who was an alchemist during their earthly life, we might make a connection with the name Merlin. This does not mean that Merlin is your guide.

All my life, Native American Indians, their culture, and their way of life have fascinated me. Over the years I have purchased many items and artefacts relating to Native American Indian culture, including books, various bronze statues and also a six-foot, carved wooden figure of an Indian chief that takes pride of place in my home. Now I know that I have a Native American guide who is my spirit protector, gatekeeper, guardian angel and, most importantly, my friend. Although he has been around me all my life, until I started my spiritual journey I was unaware of his existence. You may be aware that you have been drawn to a certain culture. This could have been influenced by one of your own guides, without you having been aware of the connection.

The Need for a Balanced Approach

Working with Spirit is a wonderful experience. When you first become aware of Spirit and start to work with your guides it may leave you feeling excited and uplifted. It is all too easy to allow yourself to become embroiled in the Spirit Realm, and the energy that Spirit brings to you, to the extent that interacting with Spirit can become all that you want to do. What has happened when you feel this way is that you have tapped into, and become fascinated with, a world of love, where there is no anger, hatred, or ill feeling towards one's fellows.

So be careful. You have a life to live in the material world. We are all spirit beings, living a spiritual existence in a physical world. Remember that you are here for a purpose. You must live your life and enjoy everything that you are required to experience in the material world: the good times and those that are not so good. These experiences are all essential for your spiritual progress. For when we return to the Spirit Realm, if we have not learned a better understanding of life, and of our soul journey, then we have not lived to our true potential.

Spirit people will happily draw close to work with, or to progress your development at any time during the day or night. In my experience this usually happens between the hours of two and five o'clock in the morning. Although it is not true to say that they have no concept of time, they do not understand time on our side of life. Time is utilized differently in their world.

Establish Clear Boundaries

The Spirit World is full of love and compassion for humanity and they will never do anything to harm you intentionally. However it can still be a shock when you are woken up in the middle of the night to find people standing around your bed shouting, 'Wake up, you're not listening to us,' and feeling as if you are being choked. Believe me when I say that seeing a pair of spirit hands and arms with no body, lifting the duvet up, can be a harrowing experience for anyone, even for the most experienced of mediums.

Your spirit guides will only come and work with you if you give them permission to do so. However, just like ourselves, sometimes they can become over enthusiastic in their work. If spirit people are coming to you at all times of the day or night, it may feel lovely to you during the early stages of your development, but this is not acceptable.

It is important that you are in control at all times. You must have discipline in your mediumship. Therefore, until you have confidence in, and a good understanding of, whatever is taking place, ask your gatekeeper (or spirit protector) only to allow contact to take place when you are in a controlled environment such as a development circle.

Being woken up in the small hours of the morning can have a detrimental effect on your health, making you feel unwell, lethargic and drained of energy. Consequently it is necessary to establish some rules and to set your boundaries. You must never overlook the importance of setting your boundaries with your spiritual workers. Setting your boundaries with your spirit workers is an important part of your spiritual journey that must not be overlooked. It is a part of mediumistic development that is not really discussed openly until something happens in your journey that you may not like or understand. You must establish guidelines concerning the kind of things that you will and will not accept, when working with the Spirit World.

Set rules to define the working arrangements that you are willing to accept. Be firm in your resolve, and be consistent. No, means No. Always remember that this is your time to live and to enjoy your life on this world. Remember, all development is an agreement and an understanding between you and them. They may (and can) approach you to work with them at any time in the day or night.

When something arises in your mediumship that you don't want to be part of, you have the right to refuse to be involved. If you do not like the feel of an energy, or if something happens that makes you feel uneasy, tell them to stop and to take it away from you. Be firm. You are in charge.

In my case, when I go to sleep at night I connect with the Spirit Realm through an energy beam of white light. When I am asleep, my spirit guides work with me to develop my mediumship. This is usually the best time for them to work with us since there is usually little interference from us when we are in the sleep state.

Remain Grounded

Whenever you work with Spirit it is most important to keep yourself grounded. When you have touched upon the energy that comes from the Spirit Realm it is very easy to allow your thoughts and emotions, to run wild. It is easy to get enchanted by the energy and love that comes from the Spirit Realm. There is no other feeling like it. Unless you have experienced it for yourself it is hard to explain. You must learn to ground yourself: to keep your feet firmly planted on the ground. Ensure that you are always aware of your surroundings, and always remember that you have a life to live in this, the material world. Remember to keep a sense of balance. Your material life takes precedence over your involvement with Spirit.

As you learn to open a channel and tap into energy, it is important to learn to close it down after you have finished working with those from the Spirit World. This is known as 'grounding' yourself. It is not advisable to leave yourself in an open state of attunement as this will drain your energy and can make you feel unwell.

An encounter with Spirit that made me aware of the need for me to establish boundaries

I think I should take this opportunity to tell you about an experience that happened to me during the early stages of my mediumship development. I was invited to join a development circle for mental mediumship/clairvoyance. It comprised of a lovely group of people with exceptional gifts, who met regularly on a Tuesday evening. In order to help us to learn how to raise our vibrations, and to help make the connection with people of the Spirit Realm, we would start the session by sitting quietly and following a guided meditation.

One evening, roughly halfway through the guided meditation, I became very aware of an energy building up behind me. Eventually it began to surround my whole body. I had never experienced anything like this before. The energy felt alive, lovely and comforting. Strong and vibrant is the only way that I can explain it to you. I loved the feeling of this energy as it slowly started to come forward and surround me. I accepted it, and openly allowed it to draw even closer to me.

As the energy got stronger, I began to shake slightly. When it drew even closer the intensity of the shaking increased, until I could not stop the ferocity of the shaking. My breathing became erratic, and my whole body began to shake violently. I could feel my heart racing and thumping against my chest wall. I thought I was having a heart attack. I could hear the tutor's voice in the distance trying to reassure me that everything was all right and entreating me to listen to her voice. After a period of time I felt the energy withdraw, and then leave me completely. The shaking started to subside, and my body returned to a state of calm.

This experience really shook me and rocked my mediumship. The tutor explained that what I had experienced had been trance mediumship. 'What is this trance energy?' I asked myself. 'What is trance?' I was not sure whether I ever wanted to experience it again, and even asked myself if mediumship was really a path that I wanted to continue to pursue.

As I drove home, I could think of nothing but the events that had taken place at the development circle that evening. I spoke to Gail when I got home and tried to explain to her what had happened at the development group. I know that Gail didn't understand it. Neither did I. However, she has always had a calming influence over me, and is my anchor when I need reassurance. Believe me, this was exactly what I needed that evening.

We eventually retired to bed around one o'clock in the morning, but it was not until about four o'clock that I fell asleep. I had been sleeping for quite some time when, all of a sudden, I awoke from my slumber and felt that same energy around me. I leapt from the bed shouting, 'Don't you dare! Don't you dare!' To be truthful it frightened me. I was on my own. There was no tutor to give me guidance, and Gail had already left for her work. Once again my mind started to race. I couldn't control my thoughts. I really was frightened.

Later that day I spoke to my tutor who asked me if I had spoken to my spirit guide and set my boundaries with them. 'What do you mean by boundaries?' I asked. This is a practical example of why it is important to set your boundaries concerning what you are, and are not, willing to accept. Now that I have a better understanding of the altered state of trance mediumship, I realize that what took place that evening was really a turning point in my mediumship and spiritual journey. It is always important to set your boundaries with your spirit protectors – I always do!

The Importance of Attitude

As with any other thing that we do, our attitude is of prime importance when working with Spirit. Spirit people are keen to work with us and to assist us in our spiritual development. However, in all our dealings with them it is essential that we adopt the correct approach. Positive attitudes that will contribute to more effective working include dedication, discipline, honesty and trust. Negative attitudes, such as ego, jealousy, doubt and insecurity, can impede our development.

Jealousy, Insecurity and Feelings of Inadequacy

Jealousy is highly detrimental to mediumship development. It is a horrible disgusting trait, a 'green-eyed monster' that rears its ugly head from time to time in the Spiritualist Movement. At the very least it can block one's own development. Occasionally it can result in one medium attempting vindictively, to repress the development of another by giving bad advice, or by trying to steer them away from achieving their true potential.

Jealousy arises through feelings of insecurity, inferiority, or as a result of ego. It can occur at any stage in our development and is something that we should be vigilant of at all times. In the early stages of mediumistic development we may become aware that our peers appear to be progressing more rapidly than ourselves. They may seem to be acquiring gifts that we particularly wish to attain.

This could be an issue also for the experienced medium or tutor, who may feel threatened by the rate of development of one of their students. It could make them doubt their own abilities, or cause them to become concerned about the rate of their own mediumistic development. At some time in their development most people will have doubts. They may doubt themselves, their link with Spirit and their ability to develop. Occasional doubt is natural, but when it becomes frequent it can lead to insecurity, and can impair one's ability to work with Spirit. Try to dispel doubt.

I cannot emphasize too strongly that one should not covet the abilities of others. Try not to compare yourself to others. At all times your gifts are exactly what they should be. Be content with your own unique gift(s) and be happy for others as they develop.

Some Observations on the Subject of Advice from Others

There are many good people on this side of life who will give you sound advice, guidance, and support during your development. However, be aware that there are some who deliberately will try to give you bad advice in order to impede your spiritual development.

There are many mediums who believe that the Spirit Realm influences every word they speak. Sadly this is not always true. I have no doubt that some of their teachings and words of wisdom are influenced by their spirit guides. However, you should be aware that some of the information given to you by mediums will be their own thoughts. It is advisable to research things for yourself, to learn to absorb as much information as possible and to rely on your own intuition.

Eventually, through the love of Spirit, you will find a group of people whose intentions are purely spiritual and unselfish. These people will have a true understanding that everyone's gift is unique, and will work with you to develop both your mediumship and their own. The mutual support that you will provide to each other, together with the love and compassion that comes to us from the Spirit World will help you to develop in complete harmony.

Unfortunately, I know of a few mediums that have become so jealous of other people's mediumship that their own development has become stagnant. Be wary of this. The Spirit World has no time for this, and neither should we. I pray for these people every day.

Ego

One of my primary, and longest standing, spirit guides is Mr. Harry (Henry to his friends) Edwards. Over time he has become a great teacher, role model and mentor to me. Mr. Edwards, who passed over in 1976, has been referred to as the greatest spiritual healer of his time. He was the president of the National Federation of Spiritual Healing and established the Harry Edwards Spiritual Healing Sanctuary at Shere in Surrey that is still operational at the time of writing this book.

As a spiritual healer, Mr. Edwards helped thousands of people from all walks of life (including royalty). Remarkable improvements and cures have been attributed to his healing, including many involving diseases that had been said by doctors to be incurable.[1] He always affirmed that it was not himself, but Spirit that was responsible. Considering how he has influenced my own healing journey from the Spirit side of life, the following statement that was written by him before his death, as part of an article that was published posthumously in The Spiritual Healer, is remarkable.

'I am therefore confident that I shall be of greater service to you now that I have passed into my Spirit life than when I was living amongst you.'

Mr. Edwards supplied this section concerning ego. I cannot remember writing any of it.

Where mediumship is concerned, ego is a terrible thing. It is negative and destructive and goes against the very core of what mediumship is trying to achieve. Everyone is equal in the eyes of the Divine Spirit. No one person has a gift that is greater or stronger than that of anyone else. We are all part of the great picture of life. We have our own special attributes, and contribution to make. It is the devotion of your love to the Spirit Realm that is important, together with the under-standing that we are striving to help each other on both sides of life. We are working in harmony on our (the spirit) side of life and we are looking for harmony to be on your (the material) side also. There are no egos on the spirit side of life. We do not have time for that. On the Spirit side we are all equal. No one is placed above anyone else. This concept should also be promoted on your (the material) side of life.

There is a far better understanding of these matters on our side of life. Anyone who thinks that they or their gift is better, really has a small, closed mind. We have no time for ego. For a short time, because people may have put you on a pedestal, you may have a belief in your own importance. However, when you come to our side of life you will realize the error of your ways.

It is nice to be recognized for the hard work that you have put into your development. Remember this though; we also have put a lot of time and effort into developing people in our side of life to bring the wonderful gift of mediumship through to your world. No one on our side looks for praise. The only one who should be praised is the Divine Creator, of whom, through time, we will all have a better understanding.
Harry Edwards

Humility, Truth and Trust

Always be true to yourself, to the Spirit Realm, and to your fellow man. Everyone's journey is unique; everyone's path is his or her own. You should be happy with the gifts that you have been given, for you are unique. Everyone must decide how far they wish to travel on their journey of enlightenment. The best piece of advice that I can give to you is to trust your guides and follow their advice. Stay on the path that they have laid out before you, and try to keep focused on the job in hand. I must confess that sometimes it is hard to do this in the busy world in which we live.

Mediums can suffer from blockages in their development. Usually this is caused simply by starting to doubt their mediumistic ability, or by being disappointed with their rate of progress. People develop their gifts at different rates; your gift can only manifest itself when the time is right for you, and for the Spirit Realm. You may try to speed things up but it won't work. The spirit people are in charge of your rate of development at all times.

A Duty of Care

You must always be mindful of the fact that mediumship is not just a gift of communication. It is a contract to be of service to the Divine Creator. You have a duty of care to the recipient of any message or information that you provide. You must be truthful concerning any communication that is relayed to you by your communicator from Spirit. Never corrupt or alter information that you have received in order to gain favor, or perhaps because the recipient may be looking for something that has not come through in the communication.

Just remember these simple words of advice. Your attitude is all-important. Believe in yourself and in your involvement with Spirit. Be honest at all times. Do not compare your gifts with those of others. Be content. Temper self-belief with humility (remember the whole purpose of this work is to help others, not yourself). You should recognize that we are all human. No one is perfect. If we were then our spiritual journey would be complete. These are principles to which we should all aspire.

Mediumistic Development

Many people, when they first become aware of the presence of Spirit, will decide to investigate the strange experiences that they are having. They will look for answers to explain the things that they are experiencing, and the reason why they have started to happen at this time in their lives. Some will seek to develop their mediumship. For those who wish to do so, the first port of call should be to visit a spiritualist church. During the church services, evidence is given to prove the existence of life after death. Usually, various groups and classes are provided to assist those who wish to develop their spiritual gifts.

Awareness Groups

An open awareness group is a good way of starting your journey. These groups support you in learning to meditate and in raising your vibrations in order to receive information from the Spirit World. Everything takes place in a safe, controlled environment. These groups are open to the public. Usually they are led by experienced mediums, or people with considerable knowledge of Spiritualism. Group members will usually sit in meditation for a period of time after which they will openly discuss any experiences, messages or visions that they may have had, with each other.

Development Circles

These are also run by experienced mediums and are the next stage up from an awareness group. Usually they are 'closed' groups. That is, they are not open to the public. Often there is a limit set on the number of members, and there may be a waiting list of those who wish to join. Circle members will be instructed about different aspects of mediumship and will learn how to develop their spiritual connection to a higher degree. Again these can be found at spiritualist churches and some other organizations. In addition, small groups of experienced and developing mediums often meet to progress their development in home circles.

As in the case of awareness groups, time is spent in meditation and in raising vibrations. However, in development circles, members are supported to form a connection with Spirit and to develop psychic abilities in preparation for platform work, or for delivering private readings. Circle members will give messages to their colleagues in the group. They will learn to become confident concerning their communication with spirit people and with the messages that they give. In a development group you must feel comfortable, safe and protected at all times. You must never feel under pressure to do, or to become involved in anything that you consider to be beyond your ability.

Help from Spirit

During the various stages of your mediumistic development many people from the Spirit World will work with you, and will provide help and guidance. Most of these people will be in the background, organizing and 'tweaking' the energy and vibrations around you. They will experiment, to determine which form of communication is best suited to your mediumship at any particular time. It is necessary to ensure that appropriate information can be delivered promptly, accurately and effectively, from their side of life, through you, to the recipient. Therefore, a great deal of time and effort will be expended in order to get things right, both for you (the medium) and for them (the spirit guides and communicators that work with you).

When you hear and start to listen to your communicator (guide), he or she becomes more than a guide to you. They become good friends and are part of your spiritual family. It is important to remember that you must be respectful to them at all times, as they will always be respectful to you. It is an agreement between them and you to work together and to develop the gift of mediumship that lies within you, whatever it may be. It is also important to be aware that they have the right to leave you at any time, as we also have the right to stop developing mediumship at any time. Just as we have freedom of choice, so do our spirit guides. The coming together through mediumship is an agreement between them and us to work on equal terms.

It is a lovely thought that your family members in the Spirit World will always be around you, and will have a keen interest in your development; that they will be there to give you support and comfort when it is needed.

Emotional Turmoil

Be aware that throughout your development you will experience all kinds of emotional turmoil, confusion, mental blocks, and frustrations. This is a necessary part of mediumship development that we all have to go through in order to learn to believe in and trust our spirit friends. Spirit people are intelligent, courteous, and are aware of your thoughts at all times. Most of them have experienced living in our world at some time in the past. You must place your trust in the Spirit World, and have the understanding and faith that your spirit guides and helpers know what they are doing during all stages in your development.

Ailments and Mediumship

As a general rule, mediums do not keep good health. Most of the mediums that I know suffer from a variety of physical ailments and health problems. Kidney stones, diabetes, thyroid problems seem to be a few of the more common conditions. To some extent this may reflect the demographics of mediums as a group. As a general rule they are older adults and are therefore more likely to suffer from multiple long-term conditions. However, Spirit has informed me that, owing to changes that take place both within your energy and your physical structure, during various stages in your development, it is likely that you will feel unwell. We often talk about having gone through 'shifts' during our development. These can feel very similar to flu or cold symptoms, and can bring forward complaints such as shingles. You can go through periods of time that you just don't feel right and can't explain what is going on. This I'm afraid to say is part of your journey. Consequently, when you work with Spirit it is important for you to pay attention to your general health and wellbeing.

Some mediums say that working in the altered state of trance can reduce your life expectancy by several years. Ten years is the figure that seems to be quoted most frequently. I believe this was a figure that was mentioned many years ago by the Spirit World. However, it is my belief that, since the Spirit World no longer take mediums to the same depths of trance as they used to many years ago, this is now not the case.

Traditionally, trance mediums have relied upon the use of ectoplasm in order to achieve physical manifestations. However this involves considerable risk for the physical trance medium. Spirit workers are always seeking new ways of working. They do not sit about idly, waiting for things to happen by chance. They are constantly making advancements in all aspects of mediumship and in the development of new technologies, just as we are on our side of life.

They have told us that they are now experimenting with quantum physics in mediumship as an alternative to ectoplasm for manifesting physical phenomena. They believe that this will reduce risk of harm for the trance medium, and have informed us that once this approach has been perfected, ectoplasm will largely become a thing of the past.

They have also informed us that ectoplasm is used in healing in the form of psychic bandages. The composition of a psychic bandage is very similar, but not identical to, the ectoplasm that is used to create physical manifestations during a materialization séance. It is a living substance that is made from various components, some of which are provided by Spirit, and some from the physical body of the trance medium. It is high in protein and is used to enhance the recovery of an organ in the physical body through the spirit body.

My Journey Continues: My Early Experiences of Development Circles

Since I had been receiving visitations from spirit people at all times of the day and night, I took the view that I would need to take action to ensure that, in the future, I was in control of my interactions with Spirit. This is what led me to seek to become a member of a development circle.

As previously stated, I joined a development circle for mental mediumship that was held on a Wednesday evening (in order to differentiate between the different groups that I attended I will refer to this as Group 1). At the time I had no idea what to expect from such a group. I knew that I had to start somewhere, and this was the first door of many that would be opened for me in my journey of mediumship. The class was quite large, approximately thirty people, who were sitting in the shape of a huge circle.

The lady who was leading the class asked everyone to begin by closing their eyes and to follow a guided meditation. I managed to listen to what was being said, but to be honest it just felt to me that I was sitting with my eyes closed. After a while the lady asked everyone to bring themselves back into the room (which I couldn't quite understand since I had not been anywhere). She then went around the group and asked certain members of the circle to relate to the others, the wonderful journeys they had experienced while sitting in meditation.

Some of the experiences seemed quite fanciful to me. These included floating in the air on the backs of eagles, sitting on the tops of mountains and speaking to spirit guides. I wondered about the sanity of the people who were describing them. Finally, some of the group were asked to relate any messages that they had received (or were receiving) from Spirit, to the other group members. This part of the evening fascinated me. I listened intently to what was being said. Some of the messages seemed to be of relevance to other members of the group. However, I have to say that since they all seemed to know each other quite well, I was a little skeptical concerning the whole process.

After attending the circle for a few weeks I was becoming aware of colors that would appear inside my mind during the meditation. Eventually I started to see people's faces, pictures, places of work, locations and events that had taken place in times gone by, none of which I had ever been to or had seen previously. I was beginning to find these images really interesting. Sadly, after just a couple of months, owing to other work commitments the lady medium found that she was unable to continue to support the development circle and it was disbanded.

This led me to seek out a new development circle. It took me a few months to be able find one that was suitable, and to be invited to join. In the interim I regularly attended two open awareness groups in Edinburgh. In this circle I met some wonderful people who, like myself, had become aware of the Spirit World and were seeking a better understanding of this strange, unseen world.

During the first three months of my attendance at this development circle (Group 2) I was taught to meditate. I also took part in some psychic exercises, learned about chakras and wrote essays on the principles of Spiritualism (amongst other subjects). Two development circles were running concurrently within this building and it was decided to amalgamate them. As a consequence, over the next three months I was required to repeat all the exercises, essays and material that I had already covered.

Luckily I had been invited to join yet another circle on a different evening (Group 3). To me, this seemed to be a far better one. (I mention this development circle and some of the things that took place in it later in this book.) Although I was aware that some tutors are averse to students being members of more than one development circle at the same time, I continued to attend both and did not inform the tutors that I was doing so. I did not care about such pettiness. I was hungry for knowledge. I felt that it was the Spirit World that had opened up this avenue for me to walk down and I wasn't going to miss the opportunity.

Just over six months after I joined Group 3 I was feeling confident about sitting in meditation. I was reading lots of literature regarding all aspects of Spiritualism. It was like a sponge soaking up water. I was now able to link to a communicator from the Spirit World and was becoming able to give short messages within the two development circles. My confidence was building and the other group members were accepting the information that I was relating to them. Feedback from the recipients was positive.

My Introduction to the Altered State of Trance

In Group 3, I was introduced to the altered state of trance (that I will address in detail later). Meanwhile, Group 2 was starting to split up. Cliques were starting to form, and a strange negativity was being felt within the energy when the group came together to work. There seemed to be a lack of harmony within the group, which was no longer working well. Some of the members had started to feel that they were better than others. To me these people had lost sight of what it was that they were trying to achieve.

One night, when I was attending Group 2, the lady who had given me advice and who had acted as lead for the first development class, approached me and asked if I would like to join a trance mediumship class that she was forming on another evening at the same venue as Group 2. Since I was already experiencing going into the trance states in Group 3, I jumped at this opportunity.

A Choice To Be Made

The date was set and I was looking forward to the new class

beginning. The following week, when I attended Group 2, the tutor asked if she could have a quiet word with me. She stated that she had been told that I was thinking about joining a trance mediumship development class and wanted to know if this was correct. 'Yes this information is correct,' I told her. She proceeded to tell me that she did not have a great knowledge of trance mediumship, but she felt that I should concentrate on the development of mental mediumship. She suggested that I should delay training in trance mediumship for a few years.

I have always believed that the Spirit World has guided my journey, and that when 'doors are opened' for me I have to choose whether to 'close them' or to 'walk through'. On this occasion the tutor required me to choose whether to join the trance class or to remain a member of Group 2. I had to make the choice between the new trance class and her development circle. I gave thought to this for about two seconds and then I replied to her, 'That's not a hard decision to make, it will be the trance class then!' That was the last night I sat under her guidance for development.

I did feel a little annoyed at what she had put to me that evening, but I was attending the other mental mediumship development group (Group 3) that she knew nothing about and, unlike Group 2, the harmony in that class was lovely. The Spirit World had taken me away from her teachings and the negativity that had formed within her group. As we often say in this movement, there is no such thing as chance. There is a reason and a purpose for everything that happens

Making the Connection

Attunement

Attunement is the basis of all mediumship. It can be described as being similar to tuning a radio to the correct frequency. In mediumship, the process of attunement involves allowing spirit workers to come forward in order to manipulate the energy and vibrations around you. This is usually achieved when you are in an altered state that is reached through meditation, or by 'sitting in the power'.

Attunement is required for the development of all forms of mediumship (mental, healing, or trance). There are a great many guided mediations available. Some of these are designed to assist you to meet your spirit guides. Others are intended as an aid to the achievement of various stages of attunement. Basically, attunement is about allowing yourself to be taken down into a relaxed state of mind so that the Spirit World can finely tune your senses through the manipulation of energy. This enables them to start to communicate with you.

Through time, and with dedication and practice, you will be able to form a bond with your communicator (guide) from the Spirit side of life. The early stages of development are all about getting to know your spirit communicator and learning to trust whatever they bring forward for you to see, hear or feel.

There are always people on the Spirit side of life who are working with you, even when you are asleep. Different teams of spirit helpers will be involved in each of the various phases of attunement associated with healing, mental or trance mediumship. Do not be fearful of the attunement stage of development. It is like the first time you meet someone, who later develops into a best friend. At first they may seem unfamiliar to you but through time a bond of love and friendship develops.

Some people are able to establish communication with their

guides far more quickly than others. This is a fact. Every person's journey is unique in this respect. Through time the process of attunement will become familiar to you, enabling you to link with your spirit guides as easily as holding a telephone conversation with a friend.

The Five Clairs

The most common form of attunement usually concerns visualization (experiencing images in the 'mind's eye'). This is called clairvoyance. Another common form of attunement involves tuning the hearing to receive communication from Spirit (clairaudience). Often this begins with awareness of ringing, or of a high-pitched noise, in the ears, which occurs from time to time. Clairsentience is the ability to feel information contained within the energy from the Spirit World (for example feeling cold draughts or the sense of being touched by something or someone). Sometimes it is possible to know the nature of a communication without experiencing visual, audible or tactile information. This is known as Claircognizance (sometimes referred to as Clair knowing). Clairalience is about being able to tune in to smells from the Spirit World. For example, sensing a particular perfume linked with someone from Spirit (or in my case, smelling pipe smoke as I entered my home when I first started to become aware of Spirit).

Breathing

Learning to breathe correctly is most important for all forms of mediumship. No one explained to me how important control of the breath is for mediumship development. Performed correctly, it helps to attain a state of relaxation and to achieve attunement.

Spirit people are intelligent. They will help with all aspects of our mediumship development, even breathing, if we ask. We must not forget that they are an energy-based life form. When we invite them to work with us, their energies blend with ours and become one. In essence, when we take that breath in, we are breathing in their energy and merging with them. We are connecting with their energy through the breath.

Exercise

Connecting With Spirit Through the Control of Breathing

The following exercise will help to calm the body, relax the mind, and to create the necessary conditions for the merging of your energy with that of your spirit guide(s). As with any meditation it should be performed with intention, in this case the intention of linking with Spirit. You should invite your spirit guide(s) to come forward to work with you. It is advisable to sit upright in a comfortable chair.

Close your eyes and relax for a few minutes. Allow your physical body, your mind, and the energy around you, to become calm and peaceful. Start by taking a slow, controlled, deep breath. Breathe in through your nose, filling your lungs to full capacity. As you do this, imagine that you are inhaling pure positive energy. Hold the breath for a moment and then exhale through your mouth, emptying your lungs as completely as possible. As you breathe out, imagine that you are cleansing your body of negative energy. (If you have breathing problems then take care not to cause yourself any distress. Just breathe as deeply as you are able to do so, while visualizing the in-flow of positive energy, and the release of negative energy.) Repeat this exercise several times over a couple of minutes, and then allow your breathing to return to a normal, comfortable rhythm.

Throughout this exercise you should attempt to clear your mind. At first this will be difficult. Always be conscious of your breath and the flow of energy. If you become aware of any thoughts, do not dwell upon them, just allow them to drift away.

If your mind starts to wander onto everyday matters, focus once again upon your breathing. This will return you to a relaxed state of consciousness. Continue the exercise for as long as is comfortable for you. In the initial stages, ten to fifteen minutes may be all that you can manage. The duration of time that you spend on this exercise will increase as you become more experienced.

When you start to connect with Spirit you might find that you experience particular feelings or sensations. For some, their heart rate might increase. Some might feel tightness in region of their solar plexus. Others may experience feelings of excitement or anticipation. Some may experience nothing at all, but that does not mean that the connection has not taken place. We are all different. As you become more proficient this exercise will become easier, and you will find that you are able to make the link with Spirit after just a few deep breaths.

Trance Mediumship

Trance mediumship is a general term that encompasses a range of mediumistic functions. Trance communication is a very direct form of communication in which the spirit person is allowed to speak directly through the medium, using the medium's vocal cords. It differs from mental (platform) mediumship in that, whereas in mental mediumship the medium acts as an intermediary and relays the messages to the recipient, in trance communication, the person receiving the message hears the actual words of the spirit person. Trance healing and physical trance are other aspects that are addressed later in this book.

Trance in all its forms is a very pure form of mediumship. It takes a lot of time, effort and dedication to develop this gift, both on the behalf of the developing medium and their spirit guides. The idea that anything related to trance involves demonic possession is a misrepresentation of the truth. This concept has been put forward and spread by people who have limited knowledge and understanding of trance mediumship.

This type of mediumship has nothing to do with possession. The people who live in the Spirit World do not wish to take over the medium's body. This just does not happen; it is a myth! In reality, trance is simply a direct form of spiritual communication. Indeed spirit people do not enter the medium's body at all. They simply merge their energy with the energy that is contained within the medium's aura. In addition to this, they are only able to undertake this blending process when they are invited to do so by the medium.

The process involved in developing trance mediumship is the complete opposite of that for mental mediumship. In both cases, meditation is the tool. The one thing to remember with all forms of mediumship is that it is all to do with 'vibrations'. Vibrations are a form of energy. Spirit people are discarnate. They no longer have the use of a physical body for it is not needed on their side of life. They are energy-based life forms and all communications that take place between their world and ours are vibrational energy-based. During their development, the mental medium learns to 'raise their vibrations' (they are taught to raise their vibrational thoughts upwards to a higher level). Think of the medium as being a link between the spirit communicators and the recipient of the information. They receive messages from the Spirit World, interpret them and pass them on to person receiving the message. The spirit communicators work on a far faster vibrational level than we do. To them, our world is dense and heavy. In order for them to connect with the medium the imbalance between the vibrations of the two must be reduced or corrected. This is achieved by the medium raising their vibrations and their spirit guide lowering theirs.

Conversely, the trance medium learns to lower their vibrations. This is achieved through meditation and learning to control the breath. The purpose is to enable subtle energies that surround us from the Spirit Realm to blend with our life force energy. When we talk about 'blending' taking place between Spirit and the medium, what really happens is that the spirit energy mixes and blends with the medium's own energy, which is contained within their aura.

As this blending of energies takes place, the medium can become very aware of the presence of the spirit guides and communicators who have come forward to work with them, particularly during the early stages of trance mediumship development. However, as has already been explained, the medium is not being possessed, or 'taken-over'. The medium is in control and in charge at all times. As they become more proficient, not only will the medium be able to feel the shift in energy around them as the blending process takes place, but they will also be able to sense the persona of the spirit person who has come forward to blend.

During their development, trance mediums will experience many different levels of consciousness. Initially they may be under the illusion that they will be completely unaware of whatever is taking place when they are in the altered state. Although this can happen, it is a very rare thing, particularly during the early stages of development.

A trance medium can, and will, have many different experiences and feelings when the blending of energies takes place. Some describe a feeling of ecstasy that can overcome their whole physical body, for others it can be a 'eureka' moment; a first meeting with someone they have been aware of for a long time. Others may become very emotional, full of joy and jubilation. For others it can be a very joyful and yet tearful experience. Everyone's experiences are personal and unique.

Trance mediumship is not to be taken lightly; it is a lovely form of mediumship but must be treated with great respect at all times. Regardless of how proficient you feel yourself to be, or what form of mediumship you are developing, it is important that you set your boundaries and ask for protection and guidance each time you sit for development.

If you are attracted to explore this as part of your development, until you have an understanding of the trance energies and are confident within your own mediumship and comfortable enough to start sitting for personal development on your own, I would advise you to look for a development circle led by an experienced trance medium.

Early Experiences Involving Trance

I was fortunate in that, when this unusual gift started to manifest itself within me, I was involved with people who had experience of trance mediumship. Consequently they had an understanding of what was taking place and were able to give me reassurance and guidance.

I was first introduced to the altered state of trance by the

Spirit World when I was attending a development class for mental mediumship. Luckily for me, the tutor running this group was also an experienced trance medium. This was at the time when I had also been invited to attend a trance development group that was being led by an experienced spiritualist medium who had been working for the Spirit World for more than thirty years. Both of these classes were very exciting and important to me. Everything just seemed to fall into place at the right time, and I felt very secure in both of these classes at this stage of my development.

The Tuesday class could be described best as a 'mental mediumship, and all other things spiritual, development class'. As a member of this class I was able to experience a wide range of different spiritual activities and exercises, and thereby to expand the scope of my mediumship. It was when I was a member of this group that I first experienced Trance and the blending of energy with Spirit. Following this initial experience, I would be asked by the tutor to allow this blending to take place with Spirit on each occasion that the group sat.

Every week there would be someone different from the Spirit World who would take the opportunity to come forward and blend with me. Some of the information that they brought forward was very interesting to the group. On one occasion there was communication from a merchant from Boston who knew the Fox sisters. The Fox sisters were prominent figures in the world of Spiritualism, as we know it today. This was very interesting for me since I did not know this at the time.

On another occasion, a gentleman who had lived in the Highlands came through and spoke to the group about the hardships he had endured throughout his lifetime. The spirit people who came through and spoke at our group were not great prominent figures in history. They were just normal everyday people and I loved the fact that they would take the opportunity to have their voice heard once more on this, the physical world through ourselves in our little group.

I also loved the experience of the trance class. There were ten people in this class and we would sit every week on a Wednesday night. Four of the members of the group (including the tutor) had previous experience with trance work. The other six had been handpicked by the tutor and had very little experience with this form of mediumship. I was one of these six.

We would sit in a darkened room in a cabinet used for séances (a séance cabinet is basically a large framed box with material draped over it leaving the front area exposed so that people can enter the cabinet and sit in a seat contained within the box under a red, blue or green light). The purpose of the séance cabinet is to focus and condense the trance energy, enabling it to be contained within in the cabinet. At this time I was unaware that this type of trance development is to develop physical trance mediumship (a topic that I will explore later in this book). I just followed the instructions of the tutor.

The first person who started to come forward regularly from the Spirit side of life in this group was a Native American Indian guide who worked with me and whom we got to know as Grey Horse. Through his own words, spoken through me, he informed us that belonged to the Cheyenne Nation. Over a few months he told us all about his past life and the way he and his tribe lived at one with the land. I got to know him very well. Sometimes he would present himself as wearing a full headdress. On other occasions he would appear with his whole face painted in blue war paint. Grey Horse has been with me all my earthly life and is my doorkeeper or spirit protector.

Many people from the Spirit side of life came forward to communicate with us in this development group. Often, they would give us information relating to who they were and what had happened to them before they passed over to the Spirit World. Being skeptical we decided conduct an Internet search in order to investigate the information that we had been given. The evidence that we found was such that we decided that there was no longer any need to doubt the information that we were given. I do feel that it is healthy to have an open mind and to test the Spirit World from time to time.

These classes were important to me in my development but after approximately a year personality issues were affecting the dynamics of the Tuesday group and I decided to leave. Once again I was left with no mental mediumship development group and I asked my spirit people to help me in this matter.

A few weeks later I found myself at a church watching a demonstration of platform mediumship. Afterwards, I approached the chairperson of the church and explained that I wished to join a development group. Some time later I received a phone call from him. I was told that a space had become available in the development group and was invited to the next meeting of the group. I was only too happy to accept this invitation and thanked the Spirit World for opening another door for me. The next Thursday I went to my first meeting of the group. I enjoyed the energy and the company of the people there. After attending regularly for a few months, I was invited to go to Ayr to attend a trance workshop with a tutor who had been taught under the guidance of the late Gordon Higginson (I have to say that, at that time, the name meant nothing to me).

Meeting this tutor really was the start of my trance spiritual journey; I just did not know it at the time. Over the next seven months I attended three more courses that were led by this tutor. A couple of months after attending the last of these trance workshops that year, owing to work commitments, the lady who was running the weekly trance development class decided that she could no longer continue her support for the group and asked me to take over from her. Feeling that I had reached the stage in my development where this would be possible, I was more than happy to take up the reins, or so I thought!

During the trance workshop my tutor had told me not to

continue with mental (platform) mediumship and had asked me to restrict my future development to sitting in the power and trance. He said that for the work that lay ahead it was very important for me to be able to build and to hold my own energy, and advised me to spend as much time as possible developing in the power. However, since I was enjoying all aspects of my mediumship development, I decided to ignore this advice. Instead, I continued as before, both as the acting lead for the local trance development group, and as a member of the mental mediumship development group.

This was a lovely time for me. In the trance development group I would attune with my guides and link into what was happening with the person in the séance cabinet. I was also helping the other mediums with the running of the mental mediumship development classes. About three months later I met with my tutor once again at one of his workshops. He asked the members of the class to blend with their spirit guides and to allow whatever they wished to happen, to take place.

After about an hour he asked the guides to withdraw and to step to the side. When our consciousness had returned fully, he addressed the class. Finally, he turned to me. 'There is something wrong with your development,' he told me. 'Your energy is not the same as it was the last time we met. It has changed. I don't know what has happened to you, let me think about it.'

I had no idea what the problem could be. I had been sitting regularly in the power and had been developing in the séance room. I could not understand what was wrong! The group went for a tea break, and when we came back we returned to sitting in the power. After a very short time the tutor asked us to return to full consciousness once again. He asked me to tell him what I had been doing that could account for a change in my energy since the last workshop. 'Nothing!' was my reply. 'No, you have been doing something different,' he said. 'Your energy has become depleted. Whatever you have done has set your development back at least three months.'

I had no option but to come clean and tell him that I had been running a trance development class once a week. 'I asked you to concentrate on your own development,' he said. 'I can only offer advice to help you on your journey, it is up to you if you want to take the advice on board or not!' I was gutted. How stupid I had been. In my eagerness to help the trance group and the mental mediumship development classes, I had hampered my own development. My development is important to me. I listened to my tutor and followed his advice. Immediately after the course ended I stepped down from running the trance group and withdrew from the mental mediumship development circle.

By following this advice I have now developed to a level where I am able to build and to hold my own energy sufficiently for Spirit to work through me. It has taken me some years to get to this point, but I consider it to have been well worth the journey. During the early stages of your development, it is important to think of yourself and your own development. There is plenty of time to teach others, if you feel the urge to do so, once you and your guides feel that you have reached the point where you are sufficiently experienced and qualified to do so.

Sitting in the Power

The first part of trance development is to learn to sit in the power. The pioneers of the past sat in the power of trance energy and developed their mediumship over many years to such a high standard that they were able confidently to take it out to the public. Everyone has to go through the development stages. This can take years of dedication; many people start with enthusiasm and then fall by the wayside.

I have to tell you that you can spend months, or even years in trance development without seeing any breakthrough in your trance mediumship. Many people lose interest. However, I must stress that those who persevere with all the ups and downs of trance development, eventually will have a wonderful journey and a far better understanding of the love that comes from the spirit people and the Spirit Realm.

Sitting in the power is an important part of trance development. It is also important not to allow your thoughts to rush off in any direction. You must have intent and discipline in what you are striving to achieve. Sitting in the power enables you to build your own energy. I will try to explain this for you. Imagine having a battery contained within your solar plexus area of your body. This is where the power that you need for your spiritual work is held.

At the start of your journey this battery is empty and must be filled with spiritual energy. When you are working with Spirit, from time to time you will deplete some of the energy contained within your solar plexus area. This is common during trance mediumship. However, by sitting in the power you will be able to recharge this battery and become able to hold your own power that is needed for trance work.

Sitting in the power is not new to trance mediumship, but it has not been used for quite some time. It has been re-introduced to trance development over the last few years and is firmly back amongst us today. Development takes place when you allow yourself to sit in the power. The following exercise is designed to allow you to experience it.

Exercise

Sitting in the Power

As they learn to sit in the power, some people like to have tranquil music playing. While that is pleasant, I do not find it to be absolutely necessary. It is really down to personal choice. Always say a prayer to the Divine Spirit asking for protection (I ask for this to take the form of white light that surrounds me) and give thanks to everyone who wishes to come forward from the Spirit Realm to work with you.

Sit comfortably on a chair and ask for the divine power (which for me is the energy that can only come forward from the Spirit World) to draw close and to encompass your whole being. Also ask that any spirit people, guides and helpers who will draw close to you do not blend with your energy at this time. Remember that this is an exercise. With all mediumship development exercises, discipline is a key factor. This exercise is about sitting in the divine power and not about blending with those in Spirit.

Concentrate on your breath (as explained previously in the breathing exercise) breathing in and out in a controlled manner. If you find your daily thoughts encroaching on what you are trying to achieve, simply go back to concentrating on your breathing. Each time you breathe in, allow yourself to go deeper into the power, breathing in the power of the Spirit World, stilling the mind and allowing the energies from the Spirit World to surround you completely. It is important not to interfere with the energy, just enjoy the experience and the feelings that the energy brings to you.

Allow those that come from Spirit to have the freedom to manipulate the energy around you. The energy that comes from the Spirit World is vibrant and alive. The feeling that you get is quite unique. When you are in the power you can only be energized. You cannot fall asleep. If, while practicing sitting in the power, you do fall asleep, there can only be one reason – you are not in the power!

This wonderful part of trance development is important. You don't have to sit in the power for hours. In the beginning 15 to 20 minutes is quite sufficient, but I am confident that as you start to feel the energy that comes from the Spirit World, you will want to sit more and more in the presence of that divine power

Spirit Energy Blending

During the early stages of my development I often heard experienced mediums refer to Spirit 'blending with you', 'attuning your senses', or 'tweaking your energy' and wondered what these terms meant. They would tell me that spirit guides would come forward when you were sleeping, sitting in meditation or sitting in the power and 'tweak your energy'. I was intrigued with this idea of 'tweaking' and asked about it on many occasions. What did it mean? How was it done? No one seemed to be able to give me meaningful answers. Deep down I began to wonder if they really knew. It took several years of searching before I was able to get an answer that I could relate to. Finally it was explained to me by my own spirit team.

It is my understanding that each of us has an energy field that surrounds the body. Commonly this is referred to as the aura, the existence of which has been scientifically proven through a technique known as Kirlian photography. Kirlian photography involves a range of photographic techniques and is named after Semyon Kirlian, who developed the technique after a chance observation in 1939 concerning high frequency, high-energy power sources and the production of photographic images. It has since been used to produce pictures of living things that are surrounded by a corona of light that can vary in color. Although there continues to be scientific debate on the subject, many believe this to be an image of the aura.

Spirit people are energy-based life forms and each has a unique energy structure. When they blend with us, in essence they are mixing their energies with our own energy, which exists, within and around us, in our auras. This blending process causes physical and chemical changes to take place within and around us.

When the blending process has been successful and they withdraw from us, they leave a little of their own energy within us. This answers the question of why, after blending, some spirit people only stay with us for a short time, is that they have a specific job to do that will enhance our mediumistic journey. These spirit people bring a quality of energy that is required at certain times for our own development and they only stay with us until the energy blending, or tweaking if you like, is complete.

Trance Blending

In trance mediumship we learn to shift our consciousness to one side. In this way we allow those who come forward from the Spirit World to have the freedom to voice their opinions freely and to allow their thoughts to be heard through us. The process for enabling this to happen is known as trance blending.

Trance blending is exactly what it says, blending with spirit energy under the conditions of trance. In order to allow this to happen, you follow exactly the same procedure as sitting in the power. However, on this occasion, you should give the spirit people permission to blend their energy with yours. In this case, as you say your prayer, ask for the spirit people to come forward and blend with you when they are ready to do so.

Some people may be concerned about their physical body being taken over when spirit people come forward to blend. As I have already explained, this does not happen. What actually takes place is that their (spirit) energy blends with our energy through the aura. It is about the two energies coming together from different worlds (their energy and your energy) and blending. The feelings that you get as blending takes place are quite unique. I am aware of a strange sensation, a vibrational change that takes place around my whole body.

Some beginners who are just starting their journey into trance development can find this a rather unsettling experience. Fear can generate a vibration that can have an adverse effect on what the spirit people are trying to achieve through the blending process. Believe me when I say that they do not wish to cause you any harm. Sometimes, when things are new to us, we don't quite feel as if we are in control. We may feel unsure of what is taking place around us. This is when fear can start to come into the equation.

The energies created when trance blending takes place can have an adverse effect on your general wellbeing if you allow yourself to come out of the blending process too quickly. It is imperative that you allow the energies around you to settle and to allow the spirit people to withdraw slowly once they have finished their work. Gently bring your consciousness back in a controlled manner. If you bring yourself back too abruptly you may become disoriented and could suffer feelings of dizziness, light-headedness and sickness. Therefore please take the time to come back correctly.

It may take quite a few times for them to get the blending process correct. You will probably find that that the blending of the energies becomes smoother for you through time. You must remember that each time they come forward to blend and work with you, everything they do is an experiment. On no two occasions will the blending of energies be the same. You should also understand that, in addition to those spirit people that you are aware of, there are many others who are working behind the scenes to make things happen.

If you are interested in experiencing trance I would advise you to join a development class where your development can be supervised, in a safe environment, by a tutor with experience in this type of mediumship.

Trance Communication and Trance Mediumship

It takes time and practice to become proficient in trance communication. The spirit helpers have to experiment, to enable them to learn how to manipulate their own energy and to blend with ours, in order to develop direct communication through us.

You have to develop confidence, both in trance blending and in the communication process. After blending you may be aware of words, phrases or sentences in your mind. Often these are repeated over and over. You have to learn to release the word(s) that you hear in your head. Do not interfere. Just say whatever comes into your mind. This is when you really need to put your trust in your spirit communicators. You have asked them to come forward and work with you. Do not doubt what you are receiving.

In the early stages it is common to start to doubt what we are receiving and to be fearful that the words we are hearing are our own thoughts. So we tend to sit and say nothing for fear that we will be ridiculed by the tutor running the class, or by other members of the group. I know this from my own experiences of sitting in development groups, but believe me when I say that fear is only a word, and when you start to get over the hurdle of releasing the words, the fear will become a distant memory. Holding onto the words in your own mind when you are in the trance state, can build up tension, give you a headache and can make you feel quite unwell.

Trance mediumship is not just about sitting and expecting people to come and speak through you. There will be many spirit people that you will never know, who work tirelessly behind the scenes. Each spirit person who works with a development group, or with an individual who is sitting for personal development, will have a specific job to do. Through their combined actions, they will help to ensure that the blending and communication process becomes more natural and gentle for you.

Curiouser and Curiouser

When you get used to the trance energy blending process, you may start to experience the feeling of your body being stretched, upwards and outwards. Alternatively you may feel as if you are shrinking. These sensations can be disconcerting the first time you experience them, but do not worry, you are not getting larger or smaller; all that is happening is that you are becoming aware of the energy around you being manipulated. You may start to rock from side to side on the chair. This could continue for quite some time. Intermittently you might stop for short intervals before continuing to rock from side to side once again. Not everyone will experience this rocking motion but be aware that it can happen as a consequence of the energies being manipulated as they combine during the blending process.

If the spirit people wish you to stand up you may find yourself starting to rock backwards and forwards on the chair and have the impulse to stand. If this should happen, the thought will be in your head and you will question the impulse to act. You will not spring up from the chair. However, you will be influenced by the Spirit World, allowing yourself to go through the motions of being slowly lifted up from the chair and onto your feet. When, and if, this takes place you must trust what you are being directed to do.

As you start to rise out of the chair you may feel very unstable. When you are standing you may be a little unsteady on your feet and could start to sway slightly from side-to-side. The spirit people may wish to keep you standing for a short while, after which they may want you to sit on the chair once again. They may want to get you to walk around the room. Usually when, and if, they get you to do this, they will only make you take a few steps forward or shuffle around in a circular motion.

Do not suppress these feelings. Usually events such as these will take place in a safe, controlled environment, such as a development group or workshop. It is unlikely that they will happen when you are alone. The spirit people are intelligent and would never embarrass you or themselves. Neither will they put you at risk when you are in the altered state of trance. Everything the spirit people do is always conducted in a controlled manner. They would never make you run around a room or have you slide off a seat onto the floor. If these types of things do happen, I'm afraid that your own thoughts have interfered with the blending process.

We often hear that people who have been in the altered state of trance have no memory of anything that they may have said or done. While this is possible, it is very rare, particularly during the early stages of trance development. No matter how deep in the trance state you may be, you will always hear the voice of the tutor who is running the group or workshop. So, in theory, if you were walking across the room and were about to bump into someone, or something, the tutor would be able to intervene and prevent you from coming to harm.

It is All About Percentages

The blending process is all about percentages. It is fair to assume that during the early stages of trance development the result of the blending process will be around five percent Spirit and ninety-five percent of yourself. You will be fully aware of what is happening, and may have a tendency to doubt the process, believing that you are just making things up. Through time, development, and learning to trust what is taking place within the altered state, the percentages slowly reverse, with the spirit communicator gaining more sway. There will always be a part of you in any communication or blending that takes place, even if it is only as little as five percent.

There are many levels of energy that the Spirit World can utilize to communicate and work through us. You must remember that we are only vessels for them to use. The spirit people will be in control of the depths to which they wish to take our consciousness. Some of the people from Spirit like to work with a very light vibrational energy. Others like to work with us in a deeper state. At all times they are in control of the energies that are utilized in trance work and in our spiritual development.

Before they can start to support you to develop specific aspects of trance mediumship, the Spirit World needs you to have an understanding of, and experience in, the altered state of trance. You must be comfortable and confident in this altered state. They need to be able to have control of the energy and to know that you trust them. This can only be achieved through dedication and by gaining experience of the blending process. When, through time, they feel that control of the trance state has been achieved, they will begin to experiment with the energy around you. They do this in order to determine your potential for further development and for specialization in one or more forms of trance mediumship.

Specific teams of spirit people are assigned for the development and delivery of each of the different aspects of trance mediumship. One team will be associated with you for trance communication, another for trance healing and yet another team for physical trance phenomena.

There were more physical trance mediums working until thirty or forty years ago. Since then, trance mediumship has been less popular. Owing to the relatively long time that it takes to develop as a trance medium, fewer people have been prepared to follow this route. Instead they have chosen mental mediumship, for which development can be achieved within a much shorter period of time. However, trends change and trance mediumship has resurfaced. More people are now willing to take the time to develop this wonderful gift of mediumship once again.

Physical Trance Mediumship

Physical trance mediumship is a specialist branch of trance mediumship in which Spirit, working through the medium, is able to produce physical manifestations such as complete or partial materializations, the production of apports, levitation and independent voice to name a few. It saddens me to say that not everyone who travels down the long road to become a trance medium will have the potential to become a physical trance medium.

Physical trance mediumship is very rare amongst the

Spiritualist Movement today, and I suppose it was no different years ago. In order to become a physical trance medium you must possess particular genetic and physical characteristics, which are needed by Spirit in order for them to manifest these phenomena. In addition, it is a long journey that requires a considerable amount of dedication and commitment from all those who are involved, both here within the material world, and in the World of Spirit.

Spirit workers will assess your potential and will guide you to follow an appropriate mediumship development path. Sometimes you will be surprised at where this path leads. I never thought for one minute I would be working for them in the field of Psychic surgery. To be a Psychic surgeon you need to be a Physical Trance medium and this has become my direction of travel. It is not intended to address the subject of physical mediumship in detail in this book. Indeed this could form the basis of a book in its own right

Healing Through Mediumship

For me, healing is the greatest form of mediumship. There is nothing more rewarding than being used for this purpose by the Spirit Realm. All types of mediumship serve one purpose and that is to heal to some degree.

Through their gift of communication, mental mediums can bring comfort to the bereaved. By providing evidence of life after death the medium seeks to let them know that although the physical body and presence may have ceased to exist as we know it, their loved ones are still there. They have merely moved on to a different plain of existence in the Spirit World. They are still very much alive and still take an interest in the daily lives of their loved ones in the material world. This knowledge can bring comfort, help to heal the broken heart and give closure to those who are grieving for lost relatives and friends.

It really is a sad time when a loved one passes over. At such times as these I find great comfort in my belief system, which has its basis in Spiritualism. Through the information that I have received from Spirit and my own experience as a medium I now know, without a doubt, that our loved ones are always around us, and that we shall meet up with them again when our time comes to pass over and return home to the Spirit World.

By linking and communicating with those in the Spirit World, mental mediums are able to deliver accurate information that only their loved ones would understand, thereby providing indisputable proof that our loved ones who have passed over are still with us, and are supporting us in our everyday lives. It is comforting to know that there are spiritualist mediums amongst us who specialize in this form of healing.

Spiritual Healing

Spiritual healing, as with any other form of healing that is carried out involving Spirit, is safe and effective. Healing energy from the Spirit World is used to bring balance to the mind, body and soul, and can help to stimulate the body's natural healing processes.

When the word spiritual is used, people automatically think of religion. However, spiritual healing is unrelated to religion. It can be administered to, or by, anyone, regardless of their religious beliefs, or lack of them. Religion and faith play no part in a spiritual healing. This is illustrated by the fact that babies, young children and animals (none of whom has any concept of religion or faith), can all receive benefit. Before the advent of modern medicine, people who were unwell frequently sought the assistance of a healer. This healer would utilize energy from the Spirit World to aid the healing process. Spiritual healing is no different today.

Training to Become a Spiritual Healer

Anyone who is interested in becoming a spiritual healer should join a registered healing organization. This will ensure that they receive appropriate and comprehensive training, and a working understanding of the necessary rules, guidelines, legal and ethical principles.

Most people are nervous when they join a healing circle. It is natural to feel like this. Healing circles are there for the aspiring students to learn, to understand the rights from the wrongs, and to be taught what is acceptable in the eyes of the Divine Spirit and the laws governing spiritual healing. An abundance of compassion and empathy are essential characteristics for anyone who wishes to be a spiritual healer. All life is precious and healing mediumship is a special gift that is granted through the love of the Divine Spirit and the Spirit World to help humankind and the animal kingdom.

The thought of healing a stranger for the first time can be very daunting. It can take time to get accustomed to standing up and having all eyes gaze upon you in the healing circle. Everyone has to go through this experience and I was no different. Always remember never to feel pressurized to do anything in any circle. If you just wish to observe what the other healers are doing within the group then that is fine.

When you feel the time is right for you, then you may join in if you wish. An experienced healer will guide you through the healing process. In addition, they may instruct you in techniques to improve the quality of the experience both for your client and for yourself. Usually the healer will ask you to put your hands onto whatever part of the person's body to which you feel drawn. It is common to start working on the back, shoulders or the head area of the person receiving the healing.

After a short period you may feel yourself being influenced to put your hands elsewhere on the person's body. If this is the case it is important to allow this to happen and not to interfere with the direction or area you are being drawn to lay your hands upon. Remember that as a healer you are only the vessel through which the healing energy is allowed to flow. When the energy starts to diminish or to 'pull back' from you, the healing is complete. Never cease a healing until the energy retracts from you. Always allow a few minutes after a healing has taken place, for the energy around you and the person who has received the healing to settle down. Always remember to gently ask the person who has received the healing to come back to full awareness.

It takes time and dedication to become a spiritual healer. Commitment is essential on the behalf of the healer. This is matched by commitment on the behalf of the people who are working with them from Spirit side of life. On average it takes about two years to become a qualified spiritual healer in which time, not only will the trainee achieve proficiency in performing the healing successfully, but they will also gain an understanding of the rules and conditions that are required by law.

As your development progresses you will experience many strange things when you are performing a healing. You may feel the healing energy as it flows. Perhaps you will get a mental image of it as colors. Some healers actually experience the pains of the person who is receiving the healing. If this happens to you, always remember the pain is not yours and ask the spirit people to take it away from you. Everyone's encounters are different and each healing is unique to you and the Spirit World. However, a major advantage of being involved in a healing circle is that when new experiences happen, there is always someone with more experience who can provide assistance and advice. So take advantage and ask as many questions as you like.

A healer cannot cure disease but has an essential part to play in the healing process

Spiritual healing is, and should always be, a natural act of healing. Basically the job of the healer is to connect with the Spirit Realm and to allow spirit workers to control the flow of healing energy that they have created on their side of life, through our physical bodies and into the person receiving the healing. It would be foolish and arrogant of a healer to think of him or herself as having the ability to cure ailments or diseases. It is the power of Divine Spirit that heals and the healing is delivered and controlled by spirit workers and healers.

We are only part of the healing process. In effect we act as a tool or a catalyst – a vessel that allows the healing to take place. A healer should not to interfere with the healing energy. They should allow their consciousness to be shifted to the side and to become detached. The further they can remove our thoughts from what is taking place, the purer and stronger the healing energy will be. This does not mean that they have to go into an altered state of trance – trance healing is another form of healing, which will be explained in another chapter.

Always remember it is a privilege to be chosen by spirit

healers for them to work with, and through us. They work together with us as a team and have the right to leave us at any time. We do not control them and they do not control us. There must be commitment on both sides. Although we may be unaware that it is happening, spirit workers make changes in and around our auric field in order to improve the flow of healing energy. They constantly manipulate the energy around us, changing and tweaking it to make the healing process more effective. These changes take place when we are working in the healing energy, when we raise our thoughts to them in meditation and when we go into the altered state of sleep.

Each person that attends for healing is unique. Consequently no two healings will ever be the same. However, the spirit healers will know exactly what is required and many spirit people will be involved in the healing process. This may include alchemists, spirit doctors and specialists in their own fields of expertise. Please remember that it is not our job to diagnose. The law does not permit this. There are many rules and conditions that must be adhered to regarding spiritual healing. As a member of a healing association you will learn the legal and ethical rules and principles, will be able to develop your confidence in working with people, and will have the opportunity to work with more experienced colleagues who will be able to give you their advice and guidance as the need arises.

The Three-way Connection Principle

With all forms of spiritual healing there is a three-way spirit connection. The spirit of the healer connects, both with the spirit of the person receiving the healing, and with the healer in the Spirit World. This three-way connection is necessary for the success of any healing. In principle this is no different from the mechanics of mental mediumship. Again, the medium must open a channel to link with the spirit communicator. In this case, information is transferred from the Spirit World, through the medium to the recipient. Spiritual healing is non-invasive and is complementary to all medical treatments. Since it is about balancing and tuning the energies around the spirit body, you do not have to be ill to feel the benefits of this type of healing.

The Importance of Attunement

Spiritual healing is no different from any other form of mediumship; there are many aspects of development you have to learn. It is not just as simple as putting your hands upon the recipient and they shall be healed. Those who wish to become a spiritual healer must learn to open a link to the Spirit World. This is essential and is achieved through the process of attunement.

In order to achieve a connection, the healer raises his or her energy. This enables a link to be established with the Spirit World through which the healing energy can be channeled by healing workers on the Spirit side of life. This process applies to all forms of spiritual healing. The healing energies must come from, and be controlled at all times by healers in the Spirit Realm. The healer in the material world is not responsible solely for the outcome. He or she is an instrument for channeling healing energies from the Spirit World to the recipient.

I cannot over emphasize the importance of spending time on attunement. It enables trainees to become acquainted with the healing energies and with their healing guides from the Spirit Realm, and to link with spirit healers. Establishment of a strong connection with Spirit is essential for the effectiveness of any form of mediumship, including spiritual healing. This is one of the most important aspects of spiritual healing development and it is something that I feel is greatly overlooked.

However, when observing trainee healers, it has been my impression that often insufficient time and emphasis is spent on the attunement process. I believe that this is not an intentional act but an oversight from the spiritual healers who are leading the healing circle. These teachers have gone through their training and many of them are, or have been, practicing platform mediums. Therefore they are fully aware of the importance of establishing a strong connection with Spirit. However, in a healing circle I have never observed the healing guide being invited to come forward. Nor has emphasis been made upon the need for time to be spent to enable the medium and the spirit healer to connect with each other, and to harmonize their energies before working with the recipient of the healing.

Spirit healers are real people. They may not have a physical body, give us their earthly name, or speak to us directly, but through the blending of energies we can get to know and feel the love and compassion they have for us and for the work they have come to do.

Most of the healing circles I have taken part in over the years follow the same process. The circle leader will begin by saying a prayer for protection to the Divine Spirit and then asks for the healing energy and guides to come forward.

As I have mentioned, this is fine if you have an understanding of the blending process with the spirit helpers. However, many trainees do not have this understanding during the early stages of their development. This does not mean that the spirit workers will not come forward to work. Like us, they have free will. They will still provide their assistance with the healing process and will support the trainee to develop the gift of healing. It would just make it a little easier if, at the beginning of their development, the trainee healer had a greater understanding of this beautiful energy that they feel and of what takes place when the Spirit World draws close to work. This is the basis of attunement.

Spirit Healers Need Training Too

Those who wish to develop as healers on the Spirit side of life must also receive tuition. They must learn to manipulate the energies contained on their side of life, to develop the connection, and to blend energies from the Spirit World with those contained within and around us, in the material world. This is referred to as the blending process. When the connection and blending has been performed correctly, a constant stream of energy begins to flow from the Spirit Realm. This energy flows through the healer here on the Earth plane, into the spirit of the person or animal that is receiving the healing.

Spiritual healing acts directly upon the spirit body of the recipient. The healing of physical ailments is an indirect effect. Since there is a direct link between the spirit and the material body, the healing of physical ailments results as a direct consequence of changes that take place in the spirit body.

My Introduction to Spiritual Healing

My involvement in spiritual healing started at a development circle for mental mediumship (platform mediumship). One of the members of the group was a Reiki Master and, having expressed an interest, I was invited to attend a Level One Reiki healing training and attunement session that he was running. Reiki attunement is about being opened up spiritually in order to channel Reiki healing energy. The process of attunement was thoroughly enjoyable and took the best part of a day to complete. I used Reiki healing from time to time with my family and friends, and found the energy to be wonderfully harmonizing.

As an observation, it is unfortunate that there is a lack of uniformity of training in Reiki. It is commendable that many teachers require students to undertake a period of practice before undertaking training and attunement at the next level. However, there are some who abbreviate the process, enabling students to progress to Reiki Master with a minimum of practical experience. This is unfortunate since the result is practitioners who are working with the public without having achieved the necessary level of training or experience that is appropriate to their grade.

I did not really do many Reiki healings. At that time I was more interested in devoting my time and effort to developing as a platform medium. The development circle involved a group of people who had no fear, and were willing to look at all aspects of mediumship. In this group I witnessed some beautiful communication that provided evidence of the continuation of life after death and we had some wonderful evenings experimenting with many branches of mediumship.

The Spirit World would show me something different each week. One week when I was asked to tell the group members the color of their auras, the Spirit Realm showed me rods of different colors, approximately a yard in length, which appeared above the heads of the sitters. I watched as the rods of color slowly descended into the heads of each of the sitters and disappeared into their bodies.

On another occasion I held the hands of the circle leader and became aware of energy flowing through my left hand, slowly ascending up the right arm of the circle leader into her body, returning down her left arm in a very slow controlled manner, and back into my right hand. No verbal communication took place between us during the exercise, but on its completion we compared notes. Without being prompted, the circle leader explained that she too had felt a flow of healing energy as heat that travelled up her right arm, through her body and down her left arm.

Experiences such as these demonstrate that there is an intelligence controlling the flow of healing energy. It seems remarkable that, not only were they able to enable this controlled flow of energy, but that both the group circle leader and I were able to experience the same feelings. I suppose these things should come as no surprise to us. I know now that spirit guides, healers and workers are always willing to experiment with us. When something like this takes place between two people there has to be the assumption that something connects us, and that can only be our spirits. We are spirits living in a physical body.

Periodically the tutor would ask members of the group to

perform healings upon one-another. Often the results were amazing and I became intrigued with the power of spiritual healing. On one occasion I was asked to work with a lady in the group. I stood behind her and asked for the healing energy to flow from the Spirit World through myself and into her body.

When attunement was established and I could feel the energy starting to build around me, I first put my hands upon her shoulders and then on her head. After a few minutes the lady slumped in her seat as if she had fallen asleep. Then I felt the healing energy start to withdraw away from me.

I lifted my hands off the lady's head and, after a short period, gently stroked her arm and asked her to come back. She stated that the healing energy felt really powerful and that it had made her relax completely. 'I will sleep tonight after that healing,' she said. At that stage in my development I really did not understand how important healing was, both for mediumship and for the Spirit World.

Distant Healing

Distant healing is the act of sending healing to a person without the need to be physically present alongside them. This form of healing is very powerful. It can be very effective for the relief of symptoms or the healing of disease (mental, physical or spiritual). It can also benefit individuals who are struggling to cope with life events (financial and marital difficulties, drink or addiction problems etc.), or those who are seeking guidance and direction in their lives. There are no limits to the things that the Spirit Realm can help us with in our physical lives. Never be afraid to ask them for help.

Healing Thoughts, Healing Lists and the Involvement of Spirit Workers

Like many others, in the early stages of my development I had no knowledge or understanding of distant healing. My first experience of it was during one of my early visits to a spiritualist church, when a lady who was taking the divine service asked the congregation to bow their heads as she read out a list of names from their healing list. As we bowed our heads, we were asked to send healing thoughts to the people whose names were being mentioned. I remember thinking to myself, what a strange thing this was to do. In the Spirit Realm there are many workers, each of whom focuses upon the performance of particular functions. Spirit people work tirelessly to coordinate the delivery of healing to meet the specific needs of those in need.

I was asked by a friend to add people onto my distant healing list. At the time I did not have one and decided to ask my spirit workers to help me to develop this form of healing. My guide told me that I was to start a book and to add people's names to it for distant healing. The following day I did this, adding the names that I had been given by my friend. I then sat in silence, went into an altered state and asked for someone to come forward from the Healing Ministry in the Spirit World.

After a short time I was aware of a spirit gentleman drawing close to me (attuning). He told me mentally to put my hand on the healing book. As I did so, I became aware of a white light that shone upwards from the book. I could see the names lifting from the pages of the healing book and disappearing into the white light. After a short while the light stopped and the gentleman from the Spirit Realm withdrew his energy and stepped back.

What an amazing experience that was. Now my list has become quite extensive, but the procedure is always the same. A spirit worker will step forward and attune themselves with my thoughts. After a while they will confirm that they have acknowledged the names on the healing list. I update my healing list on a regular basis. It brings me great comfort to know that healing energy is sent to the people who are in need, but who are unable to attend one of my healing clinics

When distant healing is sought it is good practice not to seek one particular healing guide to come forward. I never seek attunement with any specific healing guide. I know that many are present to carry out the work, so I attune my thoughts to the Spirit World and allow them to decide who the best person is to action the request for healing. Having attuned your thoughts to the Spirit World for distant healing and connected with a spirit worker you should merely give the name of the person concerned and their ailment, if it is known to you. This is sufficient for the spirit worker to initiate healing. Repetition of the same information is unnecessary.

Here is an example of spirit intelligence in distant healing. A friend sent me a request for healing for a lady in London. She had visited the Harry Edwards Sanctuary and had received healing for a cancerous condition. My friend had only told me her first name and asked for her to be added to my healing list. I added this lady's name to the list and proceeded to sit in the power for distant healing.

After a short while I became attuned with a healer. I thought of the lady's name and proceeded to ask for spiritual healing to be sent to her. As I felt the energy of the spirit healer step back, there was a period of emptiness in my mind. I received no acknowledgement that they my thoughts regarding this lady had been heard. After a short period of time the spirit healer returned to tell me that he had found her. This is how real these people on the Spirit side of life have become to me. They are involved in all aspects of my everyday life.

How does distant healing work, and what if the recipient is unaware that their name has been put forward?

Often I am asked how healing works. One question that arises frequently is how distant healing can work if the intended recipient is unaware that their name has been put forward. Following discussion with my team of spirit healers this is what I understand to happen.

When a request for healing has been made, the healer will add the name of the person to his or her distant healing list. The healer will then attune himself to the energy from the Spirit World. All relevant details regarding the person who is in need of healing will be received, and acted upon accordingly, by a spirit worker who is associated with the Healing Ministry in the Spirit World. The information will be passed through the correct channels of command, and a spirit healer, or team, will be designated to visit the person for whom the healing or assistance has been requested.

The designated spirit healer, or team of healers, communicates directly with the spirit of that person (not the physical person), and requests permission for the healing to take place. It is the spirit of the intended recipient that decides whether or not to accept the healing. There may be a reason why the spirit of that person does not want the healing to take place. Perhaps the condition or ailment that the person is suffering is an essential part of that person's spiritual journey, or important learning may be involved. Spirit healers must abide by the decision that is given by the spirit of the intended recipient. The procedure is no different whether or not distant healing takes place with the knowledge of the recipient. Everyone is treated similarly. We are all equal in the eyes of Divine Spirit.

You should never consider that any healing that does not appear to have delivered the desired result has been a failure. Many factors are involved in a healing, of which we have no understanding. Although the desired outcome may not seem to have been achieved, it may be that, following discussion with the spirit of the recipient, an alternative result may have been agreed. Always remember that we are only the connection that allows the link to form between the two worlds. Our part in the process is to attune properly, to pass on the relevant information, and to allow those in Spirit to do their work.

If distant healing is so successful, why do people need to visit a healer for treatment?

This is another question that I am commonly asked. Distant healing is a powerful, effective and convenient form of spiritual healing. Far more people will receive help from distant healing than a healer (on this side of life) will ever have the pleasure of working with directly in his or her lifetime. The reason that some people must visit a healer is that, owing to the physical composition of the healer who is working on the material side of life, they are able to donate certain qualities to the healing process that cannot be reproduced or manufactured on the spirit side of life. These qualities will assist the healing process, and are necessary for the delivery of some aspects of healing. This is the reason that some people need to visit a healer on our side of life.

Travelling with Spirit to Heal

I was awakened one morning sometime between two and six o'clock by my main control, Mr. Harry Edwards, who asked if I would like to travel with him and assist in the delivery of a healing. I immediately replied, 'Yes.' I sat upright at the side of my bed, composed myself briefly for a moment and then started to attune myself into an altered state. I was aware of Mr. Edwards slowly moving away from me in a gliding motion. He turned his head around towards me and said, 'Catch up, my boy.' Although I knew that my physical body was in my bedroom, I became aware of my spirit body rising from my physical body. This in itself was, and still is, an amazing experience. I then started to glide effortlessly in the direction that Mr. Edwards was travelling.

'What a privilege,' I thought as I found myself travelling alongside this truly gifted healer. He proceeded to tell me that, just as it had been for himself when he had been living in the physical world and practicing distant healing, through time, those receiving distant healing from me would be aware of my presence alongside them when these healings were taking place.

I had been asked to send distant healing to a lady living in England, who was a working medium. She had suffered from an attack of viral meningitis, which had left her with a multitude of complications. Although I did not realize it at the time, Mr. Edwards and I were travelling to the home of this lady.

As we entered a bedroom, I recognized the lady as soon as I saw her face. Standing around her bed were other spirit guides. This lady had also been receiving distant healing from two other trance healers. I know each of these healers well and am aware of whom their healing guides are.

Barry, a trance healer from London, works with a guide called Sam whom I had met before. Sam is a huge black gentleman from South Carolina. White Feather, a North American Indian, is the healing guide of a lovely trance healer called Irene who lives in Switzerland.

Mr. Edwards directed me to stand at the left shoulder of the lady who was about to receive the healing. He stood opposite me, at her right shoulder. Alongside Mr. Edwards there was a spirit gentleman who was dressed in Victorian clothes and looked like a doctor. Sam stood next to him. White Feather, wearing full headdress and pure white buckskins, stood proud opposite Sam. Alongside him was another spirit healer who looked very similar in his appearance to the gentleman in Victorian clothes.

The six of us formed a circle around the bed with the lady in the center. Just to set your mind at rest, when a healing such as this takes place we never see the naked body of the person who is receiving the healing. All healings are conducted with the greatest of respect and courtesy to the recipient of the healing.

Mr. Edwards asked me to watch what the others were doing, and to follow their lead. Everyone raised their arms and put their hands forward, above the lady who lay sleeping on her bed. For a few minutes we all stood like this, with our hands hovering just a few inches over the top of the lady's body. We then proceeded to raise our arms upwards. As we did so, I saw the lady's spirit body slowly rise from her physical body. When it was approximately two feet above her physical body it hovered there. The lady lay on her bed, not moving a muscle. She seemed to be in an hypnotic state. I watched with amazement as, after two or three minutes, the lady's spirit body suddenly become transparent, and energy, in the form of white pulsating lights, varying in intensity, started to flow in waves through it.

You may have seen nature programs about the strange creatures that live deep in the ocean where there is no light, which produce waves of pulsating light within their own bodies. This is the best way to describe what I was seeing as the energy flowed through this lady's spirit body. I cannot say for certain how long this phenomenon lasted, perhaps ten to fifteen minutes. When the flow of energy ceased, we then lowered our arms towards her physical body and I watched as the spirit body of the lady slowly descended and combined with her physical body. Mr. Edwards explained that the healing energy had been transferred from the Spirit side of life, into the spirit body of a person on our side of life.

What a privilege it was to have been allowed to participate in this a truly life changing experience under the guidance of these spirit healers. I took one last look at the spirit healers around the bed before gently leaving the lady's room and returning to my home in a white greyish mist. On my arrival back in my bedroom I felt myself returning to my physical body and slowly brought myself out of the altered state. Once I had becoming fully aware of my surroundings, I returned to my bed and went back to sleep.

Spirit guides or controls can come to work with you at any time of the day or night. Often I am woken in the early hours of the morning and asked to visit someone who is in need of healing. Frequently I find myself at the side of my bed, performing operations under the direction of my spirit team on someone that is not physically present. Wherever in the world they are, I am with them in my spirit form, working to heal their aliment. Through time this has become something my wife and I have accepted. Now we take it as second nature.

Awareness of the presence of the healer by the person receiving the healing or their close relatives during distant healing

On another occasion a lady asked me if I would link with my guides to see what was happening with her father. Again he was suffering from a form of meningitis. The gentleman had contracted bacterial meningitis, had become very ill and confused, and was on life support in hospital. The doctors had put him into an induced coma to help stabilize his condition. Periodically he had been brought out of the induced coma.

Initially he would respond very well but then he would relapse.

On one of these occasions he had suffered a small seizure, on others he had become very aggressive and tried to rip out the tubes that the hospital doctors had inserted into his body. He would become so confused and stressed that the hospital doctors would have no other alternative but to sedate him once again. By linking with my guides and relaying the information that I received to her, I was able to provide the lady with insight into what was happening concerning her father's condition.

As an initial piece of evidence, I was able to tell her where her father's bed was in the hospital room, how many beds were in the room and some information regarding another gentleman who was in the same ward. This helped to confirm that I had established a link through my guides, with the gentleman in question. I was also able to relate certain specifics about her father and what was happening to him.

I informed her that the spirit people were talking to her father while he was in the induced coma. They were trying to explain what had happened to him, and what the hospital doctors were trying to do to help him with his condition, on the physical side of life. On a number of occasions I was allowed to observe the spirit healers working with him. Sometimes I was permitted to assist in spirit operations.

The Doctors and Surgeons on both sides of the two worlds worked very hard with this gentleman and eventually he was fit enough to be discharged from the hospital. He is still recovering today. Significantly, he has related to his family that during the time when he was in a coma he was aware of people speaking to him, trying to explain to what had happened to him and why he was in hospital.

This corresponded with the information that was relayed by Spirit through myself to the gentleman's daughter. The strangest thing is that the gentleman's daughter told me that her father had asked members of his family, and the hospital doctors, about a

Scottish man who kept visiting him, and whom he had often seen standing at the foot of his hospital bed. How right Mr. Edwards was when he told me that people would be aware of my presence during distant healing!

Children are innocent, and it saddens me when they have an ailment that causes them pain. Throughout my spiritual healing journey, I have been privileged to work with many children who have been suffering from a variety of ailments. One particular young girl, whom I shall speak of in more detail in another chapter, is a regular visitor to one of my monthly clinics.

Kerry suffers with Crohn's disease and her mother constantly updates me regarding her condition. I often send distant healing to Kerry and her mother always seems to know when the healing has taken place. Whenever she is aware that I have been working with her daughter she will send me a text. So far she has always been correct.

On many occasions I have had the privilege to be able to astral travel with my spirit team to visit people who have requested a healing. Each time this happens I consider it to be an honor for me to be allowed to attend and to be given insight into the workings of the healing side of the Spirit Ministry. It is a healing ministry, where everyone works together in harmony.

Trance Healing

I had reached a stage in my development at which I was familiar with sitting in the power and the altered state of Trance. I had also started to investigate Spiritual and Reiki healing, and had bought a few books on each of these subjects. However, I had never heard of trance healing.

When I first heard about the subject, I searched the Internet to try to find an explanation and to gain an understanding as to what it was all about. I found information concerning trance healers and the kind of results that had been achieved through this form of mediumship. Although this was intriguing, I could find nothing specific concerning the process for delivering a trance healing. I extended my search to books and magazines, but still, I was unable find anything to describe or to explain this strange form of healing, to my satisfaction.

I found books on psychic surgeons from the Philippines who, while they were in an altered state of trance, seemingly performed spirit operations, by reaching inside the physical body of their patients and pulling out damaged or diseased body tissues and growths. I also found some books concerning psychic surgeons who worked in Great Britain and who performed non-invasive psychic surgery. At the time I could not relate to this at all.

There was a limited amount of material concerning wonderful results that had been achieved by spirit surgeons and doctors while working through some talented mediums on this side of life. However, there was nothing to explain what took place during the healing sessions, or the process used by these mediums to develop this special gift.

The problem was that the only information that I could find on the subject of trance healing concerned great pioneers of the Spiritualist Movement, and it was quite old. It was written about them after they had developed this remarkable gift and had been working with it for many years. Although reference was made in some of the books to particular events that took place in the early stages of their development, I could find no detail concerning the process used by them to develop this remarkable gift of trance healing.

Thus, I was left with yet more questions. How could I learn more about this type of healing and what it involves? Was there anyone that would be able to explain it to me more fully and, most importantly, who would teach me?

The Spirit World is dynamic. Those who dwell and work in the Spirit side of life are constantly working to develop novel medical technologies and methods to heal the sick, and to provide guidance to those who dwell in our physical world.

Consider this – there are far more people living in the Spirit Realm than there are living in our world. These people are as much alive as when they were living in our physical world. On the Spirit Plane they continue to work, seeking new knowledge and understanding and investigating techniques and technologies in order to progress both their own, and our development.

I wonder if you have ever given any thought to where the 'eureka moments' that some people have, come from? I like to think that many of the inventions and advances that happen in our physical world, have their origin with those in the Spirit World, who have passed them on to us in order to guide and support our development.

For each of us there is a pathway that is laid out before us. It is our choice whether or not to follow it. If we wish to do so, then we must simply trust and wait. We can only develop and progress at a rate that is appropriate, both for us and for those working with us in the Spirit World. No matter how you may try to increase your rate of progress, things will only happen when the time is right, both for you and for the Spirit Realm.

You cannot, and will not, have anything that is not meant to be. The guides and workers of the Spirit World are in control of your mediumship at all times. It is them that develop your mediumistic gifts, which I must say, takes time and lots of effort both by you and them. I truly believe that throughout my journey, my friends in the Spirit Realm have guided me. I have trusted Spirit, and have allowed my spiritual progression to be influenced by their thoughts and ideas. I always will.

Trance Healing Procedure

In this section I describe the standard procedure that I use for delivering a trance healing and include some advice and cautions. However, as I have already stated, it is important to remember that since every client is unique, each healing will be different. It is important not to be rigid in your approach to the healing session. Be dynamic and consider your client as an individual. For example, it could be very distressing to a person with breathing difficulties if you asked them to take deep, deep breaths. Let them breathe as deeply as they feel comfortable to do so.

Trance healing can be administered to a person either when they are seated in a chair or lying on a massage table, or bed. It is just a matter of personal choice. I prefer to perform treatments with the client lying on a massage table. I feel that it helps them to relax more easily, thus making it easier to deliver the healing. For the same reason, I also like to have relaxing music playing in the background. I place a pillow under their head and another in the hollow under their knees. I have a blanket available and ask whether they wish to be covered. As I say, it's all a matter of personal preferences.

When a healing is about to commence, I usually sit in a comfortable position at the end of the massage table alongside the client's head. I begin the healing session by saying a prayer for protection and ask to be used as the best possible channel to support the spirit healers in their work. I then wait for few minutes for the energy to settle. When I sense that this is the case, I ask my client to take three slow, deep breaths and then to return their breathing to normal. This allows them to attain a relaxed state and is the first stage in the development of the three-way connection that I referred to previously in the section on spiritual healing.

Remember the Importance of Forming the Three-way Connection

I must emphasize the importance of this three-way connection. If you fail to connect, both with the spirit of the person who has come to receive the healing and with those in Spirit, then no healing will take place! All you will do during the course of the healing is to transfer some of your own energy to the person on the table. They may feel energized immediately after the healing session, but no healing will have taken place. You will have depleted your own energy and the client will receive no lasting benefit. This is why it is imperative to make the right connection between you, the Spirit Realm and the person who is seeking help. This three-way (triangular) connection is the basis of all spiritual healing.

I ask then for a spirit healer to come forward to blend with me when they are ready. For me this happens very quickly. As I breathe in, I find my consciousness slowly drifting to the side; it is almost like falling asleep. After a couple of slow, deep breaths the blending process has taken place. Perhaps you may find that in your case this process takes longer. If so, do not let this concern you. Each of us is different and there is no one formula that applies to all.

As I have already mentioned, it is a misconception that when you are in the altered state of trance you will be unaware of your surroundings and the events that are taking place. You do not have to be in a deep somnambulistic state to be entranced.

There may be times when this will happen, but certainly it will not be the case on all occasions. Each healer who comes forward to work through you will bring their own energy and will require you to attain a particular depth of consciousness for them to work through you. Sometimes the trance state will be very light. At first this can feel strange, almost as if you are awake with your eyes closed. Other spirit healers may prefer to work with you in a deeper state of trance. It is not for us to interfere but to allow them to do the work they have arrived to do.

Don't Rely upon Receiving a Calling Card

It is too easy for us to look for a calling card from a spirit worker as they come forward. By this I mean that during the process of blending with them you may be aware of a particular sensation (a feeling, an image or a smell). Believe me when I say this is not good practice for any form of mediumship.

When they first work with you, some spirit people may use a calling card to make you aware of who it is that is coming forward during the blending process. However, with time they may no longer feel the need to announce their presence and the particular sensation that you have come to associate with them will no longer occur as they blend. Early in your journey this can be disconcerting but it does not mean that blending has not been achieved. Learn to trust.

Another reason not to rely upon calling cards is that, during the course of a healing, there can be many healers who can come forward to blend with and work through you. Each will have a specific job to do and they may, or may not wish to announce who they are. Throughout my development I have placed my trust in everyone who has wished to come forward and to work through me. As they work with me, no matter how strange the energy that they bring to me may feel, or the events that I experience, may seem, I do not interfere.

On several occasions I have found myself standing alongside

my physical body, watching myself working on a person who has come for a healing. Sometimes, as the healing takes place I can find myself looking at the back of a room, in the opposite direction from the person who is receiving the healing.

Occasionally I am no longer conscious of being present in the room. From time-to-time I may find myself walking along a beach, or sitting alongside a guide or spirit helper, having a discussion. This may be about the healing that is taking place, or just about things in general. Please understand that if experiences such as these happen to you, at all times you are completely safe and your consciousness will return once they have completed whatever task it is that they are undertaking.

Once the blending process has taken place and I have made myself available for Spirit to work through me, I do not attempt to do anything. I just allow them to work in whatever way they wish. They usually begin by lifting my hands onto the person's head, and after a short period of time I feel energy (in the form of a vibration) flowing through my body and out from my hands. I am also aware of colors that seem to flow through my body and into that of the person who is receiving the healing.

My guides have made me aware that whenever a healing takes place it is not just one spirit healer that is involved, but many people from the Spirit side of life. Several healers may be involved during a single healing session. Other spirit people will be responsible for organizing that the person in need of healing attends the correct healer, for assembling all the spirit healers that will be required to be present and for acting as observers as the healing takes place.

Although it may seem strange, I have been made aware that all healers in the Spirit Realm require to be trained. They must learn how to transfer energy from their world, through themselves, and how to blend with our own energies, here in the material world.

I have experienced this first hand; let me explain. A healing took place one day at one of my clinics. When the spirit healer had finished delivering the healing I felt his energy starting to retract from me. It felt as though he had stepped to the side. I then became aware of another spirit gentleman who came forward and started to blend with my energy.

I was aware that this gentleman was taking a good, long look at what the other gentleman had done. It was as if he had stepped forward to examine the work of the healer. I then became aware that a conversation was taking place between the two spirit people. (Which I must say is another thing that can happen in your development. Sometimes the healer will speak directly to you when performing a healing. It may be in relation to the person receiving the healing or just simply, to tell you that you are interfering with the connection. If the latter is the case please allow your conscious mind to step to the side.)

After they had spoken for a short time, the second gentleman from spirit (whom I shall call the supervisor) retracted his energy, and stepped to the side. The spirit healer then blended with me once again, addressed whatever it was that had been brought to his attention, and after a few minutes, once again retracted his energy. To me, this shows that there is spirit intelligence and a duty of care to the person who is receiving the healing.

There are spirit people whose job it is to examine the person who presents himself or herself for healing, and to determine the specific ingredients that require to be administered to them during the course of the healing. It is their job to combine the necessary energy (which we see as colors), together with whatever else may be required to address the person's problem. This is why so many people report being aware of seeing colors during a healing.

The spirit healers have explained to me that that there are certain elements within the makeup of healers on our side of life that they are unable to reproduce in the Spirit World. This is why it is essential for them to work through healers here in the material world. Healers on our side of life have an essential role in the healing process.

For me, the trance healing process starts with the energy being transferred through my hands to head of the person on the table. From here it travels through their physical body before working upon their spirit body (or soul) that is contained within their physical body. Although this is how my people start a session, yours might work differently. The energy and vibration will be very similar but the process may be different (for example they may choose not to start the session by working on the client's head). Usually after a short time has been spent working via the client's head, they will cause me to stand up and move to one side of the massage table.

I must say this can be a strange feeling. I become aware of having moved from the seat. My body feels heavy and my movements, clumsy. Until you get used to it, this can be somewhat disorienting. If ever you should have this sort of experience, the most important thing to remember is not to interfere. No matter how strange it feels to you. You can use the side of the table to steady yourself if you wish and if you feel the need to open your eyes, then that is all right too. Just remember to take deep breaths and to re-establish the connection before proceeding with the trance healing session.

Allow your arms and hands to extend out from your body so that they to hover above the physical body of the person who is receiving the healing. It is not necessary for your hands to be in contact with your client for the healing to be successful. The transference of healing energy will take place equally well whether or not there is physical contact. The healing takes place on the spirit body of your client. The spirit body is a duplicate of the physical body. Any ailments that affect the physical body are duplicated within the spiritual body. Therefore, correction of the ailment in the spirit body can help to correct the physical problem.

The placement of the hands and the decision whether or not to make physical contact is a matter of personal choice for the spirit healer. Spirit workers are intelligent, sensitive and caring people and will never do anything inappropriate. Problems only arise when the healer on this side of life interferes, so stay out of the connection! Some clients will consider any form of physical contact to be unacceptable. It is essential that you adhere to their wishes in this matter. Make sure that you seek their permission before the start of the session and in all cases it is imperative to avoid contact with any private areas. I leave it up to the healer that comes forward, but I am aware that usually I work with my hands approximately 18 inches above the client.

When the spirit people have finished performing the healing, allow them to step back gently from your energy and bring your consciousness back to within the room. It is not important to try to make your way back to the chair while you are in the trance state. Once you feel that you have returned completely, you should gently bring your client back. They may be a little disorientated at first and can often feel as if they are floating, so give them the time to slowly return to normal. Remember that everyone is different.

Trance and Trance Healing from the Perspective of Spirit

My spirit guides gave the material that is included in this section to me when I was in the altered state of trance. It explains the process from their perspective.

Each time you sit for trance, it is important to remember that each blending that takes place is an experiment. Every time you ask us to come forward, we come with the intent of working through you, the vessel. There can be many factors that inhibit us from getting it right. You can be unwell, sick or it may simply be that you have an overactive mind, which will not settle.

It is a very thin line between blending with you effectively and failure of the process due to interference from you. It is quite easy for you to allow the blending process to begin and then for you to start to interfere with it by bringing in your own ideas as to what and how things should happen. This is not what we wish to happen during the process of blending with you, but we do understand that this is common during the early stages of your development.

Your job is to allow us to take control of the energy; to trust in us, and the work we wish to achieve by working through you. This applies to all trance work. When the blending process has taken place and you are in the altered state of trance there will always be a part of you present. You will always be aware of us, and will always be able to hear our thoughts.

It is important that you listen when we speak to you. When the blending takes place and our thoughts are in your mind, you should speak the words that we impress upon you. Once you have started to speak, we will take over and continue to speak through you. Let this happen and try not to interfere. Allowing us to speak in this way is an important part of your development. Unless you allow this to happen we will not be able to say what we want to say, or to pass on advice to your world about how things can be improved with help from our side.

When we speak through you, it is not always our intention to speak about your world as we see it, and about how we can help to bring about improvements. It is sometimes just about saying, 'Hello, I am alive. How's Mrs. Jones?' People who sit for development often forget this. However, we can, and often will, speak for hours on subjects that fascinate us concerning your world and ours.

Ours is the world of the discarnate, in which we have no use for a physical body. We still have the ability to manifest a body shell if we need one, and often do so when we are visiting a séance in your world. However, this is not necessary for us to send our words and thoughts directly to someone in your world.

There is much anticipation amongst us concerning what will be achieved in the near future through physical trance mediumship, as a consequence of the work that has been put into its development by those that have been involved from both our worlds.

Physical trance mediums are rare. They carry a powerful energy that not every medium has within them. They have a particular physical composition that allows energy to be manipulated by alchemists from our side of life in order to create different types of manifestations such as materializations, independent voice, apports, etc. Psychic surgeons are physical trance mediums.

Trance healers are trance mediums that work with spirit doctors (healers) to deliver healing to those in need of help. The trance healer is able to blend with the spirit doctor and to establish a three-way connection of spirit involving themselves, the spirit doctor and the person who is in need of healing. This three-way connection takes time to perfect but it is an essential part of the healing process. After this connection has been established, the spirit doctor works directly with the spirit body of the person who is seeking help for ailments that may be affecting their physical body, mind, or spirit.

There are many more elements to a healing than just the connection of spirit. There is the intent of the trance medium to allow us to come forward in order to carry out our work. When this has been established, the trance medium becomes a battery – a generator that allows other spirit doctors and healers to connect into the trance medium's energy.

The energy flows like a current around the person who is receiving the healing. This energy is very powerful and must be treated with caution. No one is allowed to join in with the healing energy unless they are invited to do so by the spirit doctors. The energy that is created is such that many spirit people are able to come forward to work with the person receiving the healing.

Occasionally, before the healing commences the spirit healers may ask, or put the thought into the trance medium's mind, for a second healer from your side of life to be included in the healing process. In such a case, before the start of the healing session, the energy will be altered in order that the other healer's energy may be included. Once the healing process has begun, no one must join in from your side of life, and no one must touch the trance medium when the healing is taking place. Touching the medium during a trance session affects the energy and this can have implications for the health of the medium and for the person receiving the healing.

During a trance healing there is a cocoon of energy that encompasses the healer and the recipient of the healing. When this cocoon is in place, unless the trance healer attempts to interfere and to reverse the energy, it is not possible for them to contract any form of disease from the person who is receiving the healing. Always, during trance healing, and in all other aspects of trance mediumship, a team of doctors and spirit helpers is assigned to watch over the health and wellbeing of the trance medium when he or she is engaged in the work of Spirit.

As they develop, trance mediums will experience many different levels of consciousness. At the start of their development many are under the illusion that they will be completely unaware of whatever is taking place when they are in the altered state of trance. Although this can happen, it is a very rare thing, particularly during the early stages of development. When they begin their journey into the altered states of trance it is common for people to be a little afraid of this form of mediumship. Many people have misconceived ideas about trance mediumship and what it involves.

The spirit people do not take over your body. Indeed they do not enter your body. During the blending process all that happens is that their energy merges with your energy that is contained within your aura. They are able to blend in this way only when you invite them to do so.

The spirit people talk through you by building a voice box in the energy that surrounds your physical body, this is a complete replica of your own voice box and then they speak through this. When the voice box has been recreated by Spirit, you may experience the feeling that the words are coming from your throat or from your solar plexus area

There is no doubt that during various stages in your development you will feel unwell. The spirit people are working with your energies constantly, making slight changes and improvements to the energy that is contained around you. Their purpose is to enable the energy within the blending process to enhance and progress your development. By putting yourself forward to do this line of work you have agreed to allow those who come forward to experiment in order to determine your potential for development and what, through time, it may be possible to deliver or to manifest through you.

Some comments on the subject of insight that we may be given by spirit workers into the physical state of clients

Firstly, I would like to say that it is not necessary for you to know the specifics of what is wrong with your clients. The spirit healers will know what is required and will ensure that healing energy goes to wherever it is needed most. However, during the course of delivering healing, Spirit may make you aware of information concerning ailments from which your clients might be suffering.

Before saying anything further I would wish to be quite explicit about something. Legally, you are not allowed to diagnose. Except in certain special circumstances, the ability to diagnose is strictly restricted to suitably qualified members of the medical profession.

Being aware of the nature of your clients' complaints is a wonderful spiritual gift that can be brought forward by the Spirit World at any time to help enhance your mediumship. However, it carries with it a considerable burden of responsibility. You must realize that what you say to people can have devastating effects on their lives, and I am afraid to say that we are living in a world today in which people are all too happy to seek legal action against you.

When organs are diseased, damaged or not functioning correctly Spirit will show them to me as being orange in color. Cancer is always shown to me as a grey color or grey mist, which surrounds, or is attached to an organ or a part of their body.

I can also feel pain in my body that is similar in location and intensity to that which is being experienced by the person who is attending for healing. Please remember that if this should happen to you, the pain is not yours, and kindly ask your spirit team to remove it from you.

My first experience concerning this form of insight was in relation to my father's brother, my late uncle, who was awaiting results of hospital tests concerning problems that he had been having with his prostate gland. When I was thinking of him a spirit guide linked with me and showed me my uncle's prostate gland surrounded by a grey mist, and told me that my uncle had cancer. When he received the results his tests a few weeks later, the information that I had received from the Spirit Realm was proved to be correct; he had cancer of the prostate. My uncle bravely battled with his condition for a few years, but sadly he passed over in 2012. He was a great man and is dearly missed by his family and friends.

I have no control concerning whether, or when I will be shown these things by Spirit. However, I find it fascinating whenever they award me the honor of being allowed to look into someone's body, to see organs that are damaged or malfunctioning and to observe them being worked upon by spirit healers and surgeons.

My Trance Healing Journey

I would now like to explain to you how my own journey led to this gift of trance healing. Through the love and guidance of the Spirit World, I had been sitting for trance development for quite some time and was attending a trance workshop. After I had been sitting for a few minutes, I started to feel the blending process taking place. As I have already stated, whenever I experience the trance blending process, I never know who will be coming forward from the spirit side of life.

I First Become Aware of a Very Special Person

After the energies had blended I could sense that it was a male energy. The energy felt strong, comforting and very natural to me, just like that feeling that you get when you put on a favorite jacket. It seemed to be quite some time before he spoke. 'Good morning,' he said. After this I don't recall exactly what he related. I remember trying to listen to what he was saying but as soon as the words had been released, they were gone from my mind. I just know that he was talking about healing and what it had meant for him when he was living in the material world, working with people and their ailments.

The other people on this workshop were all at different levels of trance development and each was given time for Spirit to speak through them. I am delighted to say that some of these people have since become very good friends to me. Each of them has amazing trance and physical trance abilities and I have no doubt that eventually they will become well known for their wonderful gifts.

After approximately an hour, the tutor asked us to bring our consciousness back into the room. To allow us to have a short break he asked the spirit people to step to one side, but not to leave us completely. Please note that during a workshop such as this where you have been working in trance it is important to take a break. It gives you time to clear your head and to gather your thoughts. I like to go for a short walk and gather my own thoughts with my spirit team.

I have found that the mark of a good tutor is that when you return from a break, based both upon their observations, and upon information received from spirit workers (yours and their own), they will give you a little feedback concerning your progress. Not too much information, just enough to give you confidence that what you are experiencing makes sense.

When we returned to the séance room the tutor took me to one side. He said, 'I now know who is working with you. I waited for him to show himself and I now I see him clearly standing behind you.' The tutor went on to say that when I was in the altered state of trance he had seen a blue light that arched outwards from the area of my solar plexus. He then told me that he had never seen this before and that usually blue light goes into the body if it needs healing.

'I am not going to tell you who this gentleman from Spirit is at this stage,' he said to me. 'That is for you to find out for yourself through the information that the gentleman will relate to you.' Although this was somewhat frustrating at the time, it was good advice. The best confirmation of whom it is that is working with you is that which comes directly from the Spirit side of life. Any information that you receive is between you and your guide and helps to form the bond of love and trust.

Once the tutor had spoken to each of the class members, he asked us to invite our spirit people to come forward once again, and we took ourselves back down into the trance energy. After a few minutes I felt the gentleman's energy blending with mine once again. This time he started to show me pictures that I saw clairvoyantly. You will always remember experiences such as this, which happen during the early stages of development. They are exciting and should be enjoyed to the full.

First I was shown a picture of a gentleman speaking to a lady at a shop door. I could not see the man's face. It was as if I was the man, or I was seeing the conversation taking place through the man's eyes. The lady was giving him flowers for helping her. At least, that's what I thought she was doing. But at the time of seeing and receiving this information I had no clear idea of what was happening.

The next vision involved this gentleman laying his hands upon many people, performing spiritual healings. I was still only seeing these things from his perspective. Although I could see the people with whom he was working, and where his hands were upon their bodies, still I was unable to see him. This was a wonderful way for him to make himself known to me. It maintained the intrigue concerning his identity, what he did on the Earth plane, and what he was still doing in the World of Spirit.

When spirit people introduce themselves in this way you begin to get an understanding of who they are. You begin to feel the nature of the person, their love, the compassion, the desire, their reason for blending with you, and what it is that they wish to achieve together with you. This makes the bending process more special and helps to build the bond between you and them.

All of these thoughts and feelings went through my mind as I was watching this man at work. Then I was shown a partial nameplate lying on top of a desk, the only letters that I could see were EDW. Why only show me the letters EDW, why not the whole name? These three letters kept racing through my mind, and then as if a light bulb went on inside my head, I remember thinking, 'I wonder if this could be Harry Edwards?'

At this point it was time for another break, and once again the tutor asked us to return our consciousness to the room. I took this opportunity to speak to the tutor and asked him privately, if the person with whom I was working was Mr. Harry Edwards. After a brief pause he said, 'Yes, indeed it is Harry Edwards.' He then asked me not to tell anyone that Harry Edwards was working with me at this stage in my development. He asked me to keep this information to myself until such a time as it could be confirmed that that he was one of my main controls.

Now, by saying this to me, what the tutor meant was that some guides and helpers only stay with you for a short period of time during your development. They are there to 'tweak your energy' and to help you to develop some part of your mediumship ability. Having achieved whatever it is that they have come forward to do, they then leave you and move on to support the development of someone else. This is an important part of development. The spirit person has a specialist job that they have chosen to do.

I could hardly control my excitement. HARRY EDWARDS was working with me! Lots of thoughts now were running through my head. My mind was all over the place! I felt emotional, tearful, scared, joyful, excited, lucky, blessed and humbled ... and then I started to doubt. 'Why me, and not someone who had spent years training to be a healer for the Spirit World?' I asked myself, 'Why pick me for healing? I am not a healer.'

Healing was not something I had really thought about in my development. I knew a little about it, but I had never made the connection. I love mediumship, especially trance. Everything about it appeals to me. 'Healing is for healers,' I thought to myself. 'I am a trance medium!'

I can now look back on these times with pleasure concerning what took place, and how I looked at things differently back then. Events such as these are to be cherished. They are the foundations of your mediumship. Periodically throughout our lives we experience key events and moments that change the direction of our journey in such a way that there is no chance of returning to where we were before. For me, this was one of those events. It fundamentally changed the direction of my spiritual journey.

Missing the Connection

The spirit people are clever people. Long before we make the connection with them, preparations are being made to support us on our journey. Here are a couple of examples. One of the first books that I ever bought concerning Spiritualism and mediumship was *A guide and introduction into the practice of Spiritual Healing* by, yes, you have guessed it correctly, Mr. Harry Edwards! This book is signed by the great man himself, and the inscription reads, 'Best wishes, Harry.'

I sat with a group one evening for trance development. Mr. Edwards's energy came forward, blended with me, and he showed himself to the group through transfiguration. All the other members of the development group witnessed this event. The process of transfiguration involves the spirit workers forming an ectoplasm mask (a kind of a skin) in front of the medium, who is sitting in the séance cabinet. This enables the spirit person who comes forward to superimpose their features over those of the medium, in order to be seen in person, by the people who are present in the room. The face, or on some occasions the whole body of the spirit person, can be seen in front of the body of the medium.

At the time I never made the connection that Mr. Edwards might be there for me. At this stage in my journey I did not know very much about him. A healer was present in the trance group and instead we all thought that Mr. Edwards had come forward to encourage this healer on his journey.

I had visited a few spiritualist churches and had received messages from the mediums working 'on the platform'. I had also sought private readings from mediums that I did not know personally, to gain insight regarding my personal development. Without exception, the mediums made reference to me as having 'healing hands'. Even with this information and direction, I still failed to make the connection between myself, and healing. I suppose that, like many developing mediums, I had my 'blinkers' on. My focus was only upon one direction of travel, the development of trance communication and physical trance phenomena.

With all that I have learned since then, I feel that I must counsel anyone who seeks to progress their spiritual journey that, it is important to keep an open mind about their direction of travel. Be open to anything and everything that the spirit people want to do with you during your development. After all they know best! The Spirit World constantly provides us with clues and items of information concerning the progression of our journeys. However, I am afraid to say that, owing to our busy lifestyles, we sometimes fail to acknowledge them.

In the context of healing it was trance healing that appealed to me most of all. However, as I have already explained, I could find no information on the process for delivering a trance healing. It seemed as if a considerable amount of my time was spent in pondering this issue. I suppose that, in my ignorance I was expecting a 'bolt of lightning to strike me', after which I would be a trance healer.

Healing is natural. In trance healing we are only the medium (the vessel, if you like) through which the healing is able to take place. The best advice I can give to anyone who is considering healing is to keep it simple. Please do not adhere to any preconceived ideas concerning whatever you think it should be. Allow those in the Spirit World who specialize in healing, to control and to conduct whatever takes place. They are the healers. The healing energy comes from their side of life. We are only the middlemen, the smallest cogs in the whole operation. Nevertheless we have a key role to play in the process. Without us that cog is missing.

If I could just give you a general piece of advice concerning healing, and any other aspect of spiritual development, it this: Always remember that it is all right to ask for help and to make mistakes. After all, we are only human.

The first trance healing, in which I took part, was at a trance workshop in Edinburgh. Although, at that stage, I had a considerable amount of experience of sitting in the power, blending with my guides, and had been getting lots of information from them, in my ignorance I had never asked them to show me how to perform a trance healing. I know this sounds stupid but nevertheless it is true. I had searched everywhere that I could think of to find details of the process but had never thought about asking my guides.

At this workshop, I was asked by the tutor to give a lady a trance healing in front of the class. Although I can laugh about it now, at the time I was petrified. I had no idea of what was involved in performing a trance healing. The lady that was to receive the healing was seated in a chair at the front of the class. I stood behind her, closed my eyes and began to breathe in and out deeply. I then tried to take control of the blending process and managed to interfere with the whole process by focusing my mind upon what I thought a trance healing to be. It was a disaster. No trance blending took place. I was left standing behind the lady with my hands resting on her shoulders and my eyes shut, with only my own thoughts going through my head.

The tutor asked me to open my eyes and then, in front of the whole group, he asked me what I had just done. 'I don't know,' was my answer, as I looked for a big hole for me to jump into. 'That was terrible,' the tutor exclaimed, 'you interfered with everything that took place and would not let them do their job.' He shook his head in disgust at me, and told me to go and sit down.

I sat back down on my seat, deflated and really embarrassed at my performance. It had been not the people in Spirit who had failed. It had been me! I had interfered with the whole process and tried to take control. I now had another fear to confront and to overcome, that of having to get up in front of a group of people to demonstrate trance healing. I knew that I would have to conquer this fear if I was ever going to be able to work with the Spirit World as a trance healer.

Later, when I connected with my guides during meditation, I apologized to Mr. Edwards and to the rest of my spirit team for what had transpired at the trance workshop. Since they work hard to get things right for us, I felt that this was the right thing to do. I was now fully focused upon developing my mediumship. I was sitting in the power for trance development for one and a half hours a day, five times a week. I was getting to know Mr. Edwards quite well and was able to recognize the feeling of the energy that he brought with him. I was also aware of lots of other people from the Spirit World who were starting to blend with me. Taking time to sit in the power and to blend with your guides really is the way to progress your trance development.

Wales, the Turning Point for Me!

An opportunity occurred for me to attend a five-day trance workshop in Wales. It was being held at a luxurious five-star hotel that boasted a swimming pool and spa facilities, and I was very excited to have been invited. The purpose of the event was to explore trance development, and to experiment with physical trance mediumship under the direction of the Spirit World.

The workshop sessions were of twelve hours duration and took place between 10.00am and 10.00pm each day. During this time we sat either in complete darkness or under red light conditions. This course was a real turning point for my spiritual journey. Previously I had no clear understanding of trance healing. However, by offering myself to what felt right to me, and by trusting Mr. Edwards and the other members of my spirit team, I had an inner knowledge that they had been instrumental in organizing my attendance at this event.

I arrived early on the Sunday afternoon and had a couple of hours of free time to explore the hotel and its grounds before the workshop introductory session. At this session, I found myself speaking to a lady called Irene who had flown all the way over from Switzerland to attend the course. It turned out that she worked full-time as a trance healer and had been working with this form of healing for many years. The introductions were made to the rest of the group and it was arranged that we would all sit in the power that evening to harmonize the energy between the group, this was to help build the foundations for the work that would take place in the coming week.

That evening at seven o'clock we sat as a group for roughly an hour. The energies that were created were lovely and the group blended together very well. It was then announced that, on the following day, the group would watch Irene demonstrate how she performed a trance healing. 'Interesting,' I thought to myself.

We met again at 10.00 am the following day. After we had been sitting in the power for approximately an hour, we were all asked to bring our consciousness back to the room. Once everyone had fully returned from the altered state, Irene was asked to pick someone from the group for a demonstration of trance healing. She chose a lady and asked her to sit on a chair that had been placed in the center of the room. She then stood behind the lady and closed her eyes. There was complete silence in the room as everyone observed what was taking place.

After a short time had passed, each of us became aware of a Native American Indian who stepped forward from the trance energy that was created as Irene blended with her healing guide. The Indian guide proceeded to lift Irene's arms upwards and stretched her arms outwards with her palms open in the direction of the lady who was about to receive the healing. 'Yes,' I thought to myself. 'Now I know what trance healing is all about!' The guide was sending trance healing energy to the lady in the chair, through the blending process that had taken place. Irene was under the control of her guide at all times. She began to shuffle around the lady who was receiving the healing. Irene's hands were always held in front of her body, pointing in the direction of the lady in the chair, and her eyes were closed.

Everything that took place during the healing was performed under the direction of her guide. To my surprise, when the trance-healing guide completed the healing session, Irene was back where she had started from, standing behind the lady who had received the healing. The group watched as the healing guide's energy gently withdrew from Irene and we waited patiently for her to return to full consciousness. This was my first experience of watching a trance healing. The only way that I can describe it is natural, beautiful and very calming.

There was another trance healer on the course, a gentleman called Barry who lives in London. Later that afternoon Irene, Barry and myself where asked to conduct trance healings in front of the group. Considering what had happened the last time I had attempted to perform a trance healing in front of a group of mediums I was really nervous. I was determined that I would not interfere with my healing guides on this occasion. I trusted my spirit team and I was aware of the need to relax and to allow them to take control of the session.

After lunch the group returned to the room and once again we all sat in the power in order to allow the energies to settle. After a short time, the tutor, Mark Webb, asked me to put a seat in the center of the room and to pick someone from within the group to act as a subject for the healing. Although I was shaking inside, I tried very hard not to show it. I chose a lady from the group, asked her to sit on the chair, placed a second chair directly behind her, and sat down. I was very aware of being watched by the other members of the group and felt very uneasy. I remember telling myself to calm down. 'Everything will be okay,' I told myself. I closed my eyes and took several deep breaths.

After a few minutes I allowed my breathing to return to normal. When I felt the blending process taking place I aware of being surrounded by the same energy that I feel when I sit in the altered state for trance mediumship. There really seemed to be no difference in the energy for trance healing. Another few minutes passed; to me they seemed more like hours. All of a sudden I had an overwhelming desire to stand up. I remember thinking that on this occasion there was no way that I was going to interfere.

I stood behind the lady and pointed my hands in her general direction. I could feel the energy flowing down my arms, out through my hands, and towards her. My hands and arms started to wave about in a controlled manner in the energy that was being created around the lady's head and body. Then I had the feeling that the spirit healers wanted to walk me around the chair in which the lady was sitting. I felt myself starting to move very slowly to my left, shuffling along with the tiniest of steps.

Although I was aware of what was taking place, I did not interfere. The spirit people managed to make me shuffle around the lady with my eyes closed, stopping wherever they wanted to administer the healing energy. Having made a complete circle around her, I returned to my chair. Throughout this whole process my eyes were closed. I put my faith and trust in them. Try walking around a chair in a room with your eyes closed, and when you open them see where you are standing.

That afternoon I took part in another two trance healings and the feedback I received was astounding. I had overcome my fears and put my trust in the spirit people who had come forward. By allowing them to take control I had finally come to experience what trance healing was all about. The tutor commented upon the way that I waved my hands around when performing trance healings. He said that although he had never seen this before, there was nothing wrong with the delivery of the trance healing. His advice was that, whatever the spirit workers wished me to do, I should just to go with it and give them the freedom to experiment.

Confirmation from Spirit of the Identity of My Main Trance Control

During the course of the week I was asked by my main trance control to perform a trance healing on the tutor who was running the workshop. For some time he had been suffering from kidney stones, which I am afraid to say, are a consequence of his involvement in trance mediumship. Under the direction of my guide I asked the tutor to sit in the center of the room and I sat on a chair to his right-hand side. I asked another two mediums, both of whom were spiritual healers, to sit either side of him in such a way that together we made a triangle formation with the tutor in the centre. I then proceeded to enter the altered state of trance and to blend with my guide.

Once blending had been achieved my guide spoke through me, giving instructions concerning how he wished the trance healing to proceed. He asked the people sitting in the outer circle, all of whom were mediums, to send their love to the gentleman receiving the healing in the center of the room. I felt my arms being lifted up and stretched outwards in the direction of the tutor. They finally came to rest on the tutor's body, in the region of his kidneys. Clairvoyantly I was being shown a quantity of stones that were situated inside the tutor's kidneys. There were quite a lot of them, all at different stages of formation, but one in particular was causing concern. It appeared to be much larger than any of the others.

Once again my guide spoke to the group through me. He said that this kidney stone was a 'tricky little fellow' and stated that he and his colleagues would attempt to break it up, in order to allow it to be passed naturally. My guide asked the group to focus their thoughts and energy on the events that were taking place in the center of the room. He explained that they were going to bombard the kidney stone with energy in the form of sound waves in order to try to break it into fragments. He asked the class to continue to send their thoughts to the center of the room and as they did this I was aware of energy pulsating down my arms into my hands and into the body of the tutor. This lasted for about five minutes, after which my guide slowly withdrew and my consciousness returned to the room.

Once the healing was concluded, everyone discussed what they had experienced, seen and had been shown clairvoyantly, during the course of the healing. A wonderful working medium called Deborah said that she had been aware of the large stone in the tutor's kidney that my guide had been working on. For me this alone was great proof.

The tutor told us that two weeks previously he had attended a hospital appointment to investigate pains in the region of his kidneys. An x-ray had shown the presence of kidney stones and, in one week's time, he was scheduled to return to hospital for further investigations and to discuss treatment options.

I have since learned that, at his next appointment, another scan had been performed and there was no sign of the large kidney stone that had been the source of his problems. It had completely disappeared.

Later that evening when we were discussing the events of the day over a coffee, Barry, the healer from London, told me that he was aware of whom it was that was working with me. He asked me if I knew who it was. He went on to say that he had known of only one healer that used the same method as he had seen that afternoon (involving three healers sitting around the person receiving the healing in a triangular formation). He told me, 'You've got Harry Edwards working with you.'

'Yes, that's correct,' I replied. Barry then went on to explain that he had worked at the Harry Edwards Healing Sanctuary as a spiritual healer.

Through Barry I was able to obtain confirmation, from the people that he knew who worked at the sanctuary, of some snippets of information that I had received from Mr. Edwards (about which I could find nothing in any of the literature that has been written about him).

When I applied to attend the workshop I had no idea that these experienced trance healers would be there. However, I have no doubt that my spirit guides did. After my first disastrous attempt at trance healing I had been searching for answers and had been sending my thoughts to my spirit guides and helpers. By arranging for me to attend this course they had answered my thoughts. In this journey there is no such thing as chance. When the time is right, everything comes to those who give their time, commitment and trust.

The Harry Edwards Healing Sanctuary

It is interesting how doors are opened to us when the time is right. Following the workshop in Wales, my new friend Barry invited Gail and me to visit The Harry Edwards Healing Sanctuary on one of the open days that are held twice a year. We went down in July. Barry met us at the airport and drove us to the sanctuary at Shere in Surrey. He very kindly spent most of the day with us at the sanctuary and introduced us to many of the people who worked there, some of whom had met Mr. Edwards when he was living in the physical world. Everyone spoke very highly of the great man, and his work.

There was a real buzz in the air as we approached the Sanctuary. I could feel the healing vibrations and the energy that has accumulated over many years. We had a wonderful day there. We were able to wonder freely through the grounds of the estate and I even found the time to sit and meditate in a small summerhouse in Cherry Tree Walk. We also had the privilege to be shown around every part of the main house including Mr. Edwards's bedroom and all of the healing rooms. We even received a spiritual healing in the main healing hall. I was so aware of Mr. Edwards's presence being with us that day. It was as if I was being shown around his home and estate by Mr. Edwards himself.

At one point Gail and I found ourselves in the main house in a bar area where two couches sit in front of a lovely big open fireplace. We sat there for a short while and I spoke about how the appearance of this room had changed over the years. I know that Gail was thinking that I was just talking nonsense. We had never been there before.

At that point two lovely elderly ladies came into the room through the patio doors that led to the gardens and sat on the couch opposite us. One of the ladies wished us good afternoon and asked if we had been to the sanctuary before, to which we replied, 'No.'

Then the other lady spoke. 'It's all changed in here. This room is not as it used to be. I've been coming here for many years and it has all been changed,' she said. Well that was confirmation, I thought to myself as I looked at Gail.

This visit to the Harry Edwards Healing Sanctuary is a wonderful memory that I shall cherish forever. Should you ever feel the desire to visit this beautiful tranquil place, you won't be disappointed. Although Mr. Edwards in no longer there, his legacy and spirit energy remains, and it always will.

Following the Path of Spirit

I have already stated that healing was an aspect of mediumship to which I had given little thought. I had never really looked into the healing side of mediumship in any depth, and could not understand why I was being chosen for this work. It took me a quite some time to get used to the thought of healing and where this branch of mediumship might lead. I had my reservations and doubts.

For weeks, I had been asking the Spirit World the question, 'Why Healing Mediumship? Why me?' One evening when we were sitting at our trance development group. I got the answer to this question. I was sitting in the séance cabinet. Mr. Edwards had come forward and started to speak through me to the group. He spoke about healing, and how important this aspect of mediumship is to the Spirit World.

He explained that it is the job of our spirit guides to identify the aspect of mediumship to which we are best suited, and the most appropriate way to progress our development. The job of the developing medium is to allow the blending process to become as natural as possible. Once you have managed to obtain a sufficient depth to your trance energy blending then they will decide the best way to utilize your gift. I could understand what had been said. It made total sense to me. It is those in the Spirit World who decide upon the direction that our paths will take, not us.

Learning To Work with Trance Healing

After I returned from Wales, I continued to sit in the power almost every day. Since the workshop something had changed. Everything had begun to feel different to me whenever I sat in the power. All kinds of different emotions were stirring and unfolding within me. As soon as I closed my eyes and started to sit in the power the colors that I was aware of seemed to be more vibrant and dense than they had been previously. I appeared to see flashes of lightning. White, silver and gold lights that would appear that were so strong it felt as if I was looking at the sun.

There would be times when I could not settle into the power and it would feel as if my third eye was being opened up. Sometimes it would feel as if someone was tickling it with a feather. At other times I could feel a band of energy around my forehead and head that would feel very heavy; a tight feeling like I was wearing a cap that was too small. I was also aware of a feeling of cobwebs all over my face and lice running through my hair. I have to say that these are not the best feelings to have when you are attempting to sit in the power. If you experience feelings such as these, it is important not to scratch at them. These are physical energies that are created by the Spirit World.

From time-to-time I would disappear completely into the power. When I was brought back, I would be unable to recall where I had been or how long I had been there. The explanation that I was given by the spirit people was that in order to prevent me from interfering with whatever they are trying to achieve, they take my consciousness away to another dimension. When at last I returned to full consciousness it seemed as if I had only just started to sit in the power. Then I would look at the clock and realize how much time had passed.

Whenever I sat in the power, I continued to blend with Mr. Edwards's energy as often as I possibly could. In this way I was able to ask him many questions concerning healing and how it works. This helped me to develop my understanding of the spiritual path that I was following. One piece of information that I received from him, which I would like to share with you, was that the healing process starts before the person arrives to see a healer.

Before requesting healing, the person with an illness or complaint will have sent their thoughts up to the Spirit World asking for help. This request will have been heard by those in spirit who will have already started work to address the issues that have been raised. I found this to be very interesting. I was enjoying the closeness and friendship that was forming through our times sitting together. I don't and never will pester Mr. Edwards with trivial things in my life but I do take comfort in the knowledge that he is there for me whenever I need his help and support.

Healing was starting to become a great part of my life. The thoughts of what could be achieved through the love of spirit, and the people that we could help with this wonderful gift of healing, occupied my mind most of the time. I continued to work with family and friends behind closed doors, carrying out healings in the privacy of my own home and learning to heal in a safe environment, under no pressure. I would love the feeling of the spirit people coming forward and blending with me, and working in the energy they brought with them seemed to make me complete.

A Change in Practice – Initial Assessment

At the start of my journey, if someone sought my help regarding a problem I never thought to ask him or her to provide me with much in the way of detail concerning his or her complaint. I would simply put my faith and trust into the members of my spirit team and would allow them to have the freedom to do whatever they wished to do with the person.

The practicality of this approach was demonstrated time and time again by the wonderful results that were obtained and the feedback that I received from my clients. Now, whenever I am requested to perform a healing by someone, I always ask him or her for a brief description of their problem together with any additional background information that they feel might be relevant.

This change in practice was stimulated by something that was said to me by someone during a general conversation that we were having concerning healing. 'Why don't you ask the people who come to seek your help for more information about their ailments and conditions?' they asked me.

'Why?' I asked.

'Well,' they said, 'whenever you go to visit your GP you don't just stand in front of him or her and say guess, what's wrong with me.'

After giving this some thought, I realized the sense behind this statement. After all, No one knows your own body better than yourself. So that is why I now ask for this additional detail from the people who come to me for healing.

A Hard Lesson To Learn – Never Attempt To Interfere

I would like to take this opportunity to tell you about something that I did, in order to prevent you from making the same kind of mistake.

A few years ago my teenage daughter contracted swine flu. She recovered from this quite quickly, but was left with some sort of recurring respiratory problem. Although she had no previous history of such, periodically thereafter she would suffer from a persistent cough. It would clear up following a course of antibiotics from the local GP, only to recur with a vengeance some weeks later. Eventually she was referred to the hospital for further investigations. The specialists found no cause for the problem and sent her home with a course of steroids that, being fearful of possible side effects, she did not take.

I worked with the Spirit World to give her healing. On each occasion she would show an immediate improvement that would last for a day or two, after which the coughing would start once again. She persevered with the coughing until she could stand it no longer before returning once again to her GP who prescribed another supply of tablets. This time they seemed to work. For about three weeks she was symptom-free, but then back came the cough.

She had been coughing severely for three days. One night, I was lying in bed listening to my daughter coughing and coughing; it just would not stop. Anyone who is a parent will understand why I decided to do what I did next. 'Right, enough is enough,' I thought to myself. 'I'm going to sort this cough out!'

It was approximately five o'clock in the morning when I went into her bedroom; my daughter was sitting up in bed. I told her that I was going to give her a healing; I then sat behind her and blended with a healer from the Spirit World. I put my hands on her back and felt the energy start to pour through my hands into her lungs. Then I interfered with the healing. I deliberately reversed the flow of energy in order to draw the energy and infection from her lungs into myself and thereby, to relieve her of the problem. I was determined to help my daughter, no matter what it would take.

The healing lasted for approximately twenty minutes, after which I returned to my bedroom, and my daughter went to sleep. In the morning her cough had almost stopped, and by the end of the day it was completely gone. However, the following day I started to cough, the cough got worse as each day passed. I tried taking cough medicine but it gave me no relief.

Three weeks later, I attended a trance development workshop that had had been arranged several months previously. I still had the persistent cough. Whenever I went into the power the cough would stop, but afterwards it seemed to get worse. My lungs felt very weak; I was coughing up mucous constantly, and slowly it was wearing me down. One morning I coughed so much that I burst a small blood vessel, causing me to bring up a small amount of blood along with the mucus. I had no option but to take time out from the course to visit a doctor who prescribed a week's course of antibiotics for me. After a few days the antibiotics seemed to be starting to help, but still I found the cough troublesome.

By this time I was at my wits end and asked Mr. Edwards for help. Immediately I felt a presence in the hotel bedroom and became aware of Mr. Edwards's energy. He spoke to me. 'This has been a lesson for you,' he said.

'A lesson?' I thought to myself. 'What lesson?'

'You must never try to draw a condition out of anyone's body,' he told me. 'During a healing you must never attempt to reverse the flow of energy. Your job as a healer is simply to allow the healing energy to flow through you. You must not interfere with the healing process.'

'This has been a hard way to learn a lesson,' I thought to myself.

'Yes,' he replied, 'it has been a hard lesson for you to learn, but it is one that you will not forget in a hurry.' I then felt a hot energy that flowed through my chest, filling my lungs and after a few days the cough resolved. He was right, it was a hard lesson to learn but it is one that I never will forget. There is no way that I will attempt to interfere in a healing ever again.

My Introduction to Psychic Surgery

One evening I received a call from a lady who introduced herself a Jane Dawson and informed me that she was a working spiritual medium. She explained that she was making an enquiry on behalf of a friend of hers who was waiting for an appointment to go into hospital to have a leg amputated. The hospital surgeons were struggling to get his blood pressure under control and were unwilling to proceed with the operation until this had been achieved.

We spoke for a few more moments about her friend's problem and then she suddenly said, 'Do you have Harry Edwards working with you?' I was amazed. Other than the members of our group I had told no one of my involvement with Mr. Edwards. This was the first person to pick up on his energy. I confirmed that this was the case. 'Oh my God,' the lady said. 'I have been asking the Universal Energy for a Harry Edwards type of healer, and they have answered by sending the main man and the person he is working through.' We arranged a date for the gentleman to visit me at my home.

When the gentleman arrived for treatment he informed me that he had undergone several operations on his leg and metal pins had been inserted into the bone. His leg was in an awful state and could not be saved. The onslaught of gangrene was imminent. He explained that he was suffering also from high blood pressure that was causing him to have severe nosebleeds. As had been explained by his friend, he told me that he was scheduled to have the leg amputated, but the operation had been delayed until his blood pressure could be controlled.

After settling the gentleman on the massage table, I gently slipped into the trance energy allowing the spirit doctors and healers to start the healing session, which lasted approximately thirty minutes. When I returned to full consciousness, I gently woke the gentleman from his slumber. He explained that, during the healing, he had been aware of colors and of the presence of spirit workers around the bed. He thanked my spirit team and me for what had taken place. A few days later I received a call from Jane, who also thanked me, and my spirit team, for seeing the gentleman. She proceeded to arrange sessions the next week, both for herself and for her gentleman friend.

The following week they both arrived for healing. The gentleman informed me that his blood pressure was much improved and that the nosebleeds had stopped. I worked with the gentleman once again. (He has since informed me that his operation was performed successfully. He is now following a more spiritual path and has started to look at the gift of healing.)

Jane was next and the healing session proceeded in the normal manner. One of my spirit workers came forward, the blending took place, and the healing process commenced. This time sometime during the healing I blended with someone whose energy felt a little different to me. I had become aware of a lady nurse pushing in a tray of surgical instruments on a trolley. The nurse appeared to be dressed in what seemed to me to be a 1950s-style uniform.

I have said before that it is not our job to interfere in what takes place. We should simply accept whatever it is that they wish to do. I found myself standing to the left side of my physical body. I watched as the person who was working through me raised my physical body out of the chair and positioned himself over Jane's head, in order to work over her face. Working on her spirit body, he then proceeded to remove Jane's (spirit) eye and placed it on a silver tray.

The surgeon then carefully performed some delicate work at the back of the spirit eye as it lay on the tray. He would reach towards the tray of instruments that had been brought in by the nurse, pick one up, use it to perform some task or other and then replace it on the trolley. Now you must remember that I am not a doctor. I was astounded and mesmerized at what I was being shown. After a short time the spirit doctor replaced the spirit eye back in Jane's spirit eye socket. I had no idea what it was that had just taken place.

At this point the energy changed once again and another blending of energies took place. A second surgeon came forward and, working through me, picked up an instrument from the tray and made an incision into what he led me to believe was the thyroid gland (in Jane's spirit body). Within a few minutes the surgery was complete, and he left as quickly as he had arrived and I felt the energy retract from me. I brought myself out of the altered state and gently asked Jane to bring her consciousness back.

She told me that during the healing session she had been aware, both of the presence of Harry Edwards, and of many spirit workers within the room. She estimated that around sixty people had been present. She went on to say that she was aware of many people working on her ailments, had felt the incision of a scalpel on her throat and was aware of surgery being performed upon her eye. After the session her eye was weeping.

The following week, in order to enable others to experience, and to benefit from my form of mediumship, Jane Dawson arranged for me to run a clinic in her home town. This was the start of my journey into psychic surgery

Some Healing Results

As healers we should never look for praise for what we do on behalf of the Spirit World. We understand that it is not us that are responsible for any healing that takes place. We are only the means for the healing energy to be transferred to the person who is in need of help. However, it is nice for the Spirit World to be given recognition for the work they carry out.

Many people who receive healing fail to give any feedback, and we never know the results of the healing. Sometimes though they will contact us and share their experiences. This chapter is dedicated to the good work that is carried out by the Spirit World and to the feedback that I have received from clients.

I have used the following cases to illustrate the kind of results that I have been able to observe as a result of the work that has been carried out through myself, by my teams of spirit healers. Some of the results fall under the category of miraculous (or amazing). Unfortunately this is not always the case. Some conditions take longer to resolve and some are never completely cured.

The Spirit World will never stop trying to help to address any ailment or condition that your client may have. Anyone who seeks help from this form of healing, either as a means of complementing conventional medical or surgical care, or as an alternative form of healing, will always benefit from it to some degree.

A Young Child with Crohn's Disease

When I was holding a clinic in Johnstone, a young woman brought her daughter Kerry along to see if there was anything that the Spirit World could do to help in relation to her daughter's condition. She told me that that Kerry suffered from a condition called Crohn's disease, which had been diagnosed when she was just over one year old.

The first time I saw her the little girl she was asleep in her pushchair. I told the mother that it is never possible to promise anyone a cure for his or her condition and explained that this form of healing complements conventional medical treatment. It does not replace it. Kerry's doctors and specialists are in charge of the management of her condition at all times. However, I told her that, if she was willing to bring her daughter along to the clinic on a regular monthly basis, I would be more than happy to work with her daughter, with her consent.

I did not want to wake or to disturb the little girl; she looked so peaceful sleeping in her pram. As I knelt down beside her I was aware of the blending process starting to take place and I felt the healing energy transfer into the body of the little girl as she lay there sleeping in her pushchair. The following day the mother got in touch with my wife and reported that, for the first time in almost a year, Kerry had slept all through the night.

The next time I held a clinic in Johnstone the mother was there with her little daughter. This time the girl was wide-awake. She was a very lively little thing and just acted like any normal child her age. At the time I knew very little about this disease and relied on the little girl's mother to describe with the history of her illness and the symptoms that she had experienced.

Crohn's disease is a long-term condition that causes inflammation of the lining of the digestive system. It can affect any part of the digestive system from the mouth to the back passage, but it most commonly occurs in the last section of the small intestine (ileum) or the large intestine (colon). This little girl seemed to have many problems resulting from her ailment. Her mother told me that frequently she suffered from abdominal pain as well as severe bouts of sickness and diarrhea.

At first Kerry was wary and was unwilling to lie on the massage table. Consequently the healing was delivered with her sitting on the table. It continued this way for the next few sessions. My wife, Gail bought books, stickers and toys to keep the little girl amused during the healing sessions. After visiting me for a treatment, the pain in her stomach would subside and eventually she started to call me 'the Magic Man'.

Gradually we gained her trust and I began to form a bond, both with the little girl and with her mother. Eventually, Kerry was willing to lie on her back on the massage table during her treatments and I passed on information to the mother regarding general things about her daughter's condition that had been shown and told to me by my team of spirit healers. She always found this information to be beneficial and on more than one occasion it was confirmed by her daughter's own doctors a week or two weeks later when they received the results of medical tests.

Whenever the condition flared up and the pain was such that her daughter became reluctant to eat, the mother would contact me and ask me to send distant healing. Being impressed by the results that were obtained, and wishing to help her daughter as best she could, the mother expressed an interest in learning to deliver healing herself. Under my guidance she has learned to open a channel to the Spirit World and has become a very good channel for the healing energies. She now performs spiritual healings on her daughter on a regular basis.

I had been working with Kerry for about a year and a half when I received a call from her mother, Claire. She was very excited, having just been informed that her daughter's condition had gone into remission. She proceeded to tell me that that she had waited more than two years to hear this wonderful news and was convinced that the Spirit World had played a major part to in the achievement of this marvelous outcome. I still send distant healing to the little girl, and continue to work with her directly, on a regular basis.

A Lady with Esophageal Stricture

A lady called Sylvia came to visit me at my clinic in Falkirk. Sylvia explained to me that, owing to a stricture of her esophagus, she had not eaten any solid food for twenty-three years. Everything she ate had to be liquidized. She told me that regularly she had to go into hospital to 'have her throat stretched' and explained that occasionally she had to be rushed into hospital to have the procedure performed as an emergency. I remember that when I worked with this lady the healing procedure was focused upon Sylvia's neck area and lasted for about twenty minutes.

The following day I had a phone call from the lady who owns the healing center in which my clinic was held. She told me that the lady 'with the throat problem' had been in touch and had made reference to a bacon roll. I couldn't quite understand the reference to the bacon roll, but I said I would telephone Sylvia later that day. In the event, I forgot. However, the next day I received a letter from her in which she stated that, since the healing, she had been able to eat some foods that she had not been capable of eating for several years.

Intrigued by this letter I immediately contacted Sylvia by telephone. She told me that I had changed her life. She had telephoned the lady who holds the clinic to tell her that, on the day following the healing session, for the first time in 23 years she had eaten a bacon roll without discomfort. She told me that she was expecting a visit from her family and that she was going to surprise them by eating a bacon roll in front of them. I cannot describe my joy and happiness at hearing this from her and, as always, I sent my thanks and blessings to Divine Spirit and to the spirit surgeons.

A Case of a Lady with Renal Failure

Jane Dawson and I were delivering a joint demonstration of trance healing and mental mediumship at a venue in Motherwell in Scotland. At these events we first give a talk about the Spirit World, mediumship, and how we were brought together through healing. Jane then raises her vibrations and link with a communicator from the Spirit World who supports her to deliver a message to a member of the audience to prove the existence of life after death. While this is happening I blend in readiness to perform a trance healing. Once Jane has finished giving them a reading we ask the member of the audience to step forward to receive a healing.

On this occasion I had the pleasure of working with a lady called Nicola who told us that she had kidney problems. Nicola settled herself on the massage table and immediately the spirit healers and doctors from the Spirit World went to work. Working through me, and under the observation of an audience of about fifty people, they performed a procedure that lasted for about twenty minutes. Halfway through the healing as Nicola lay on the massage table, several of the audience members started to cough constantly and some had to leave the room.

During a demonstration of trance healing it seems as though there is a build-up of healing energy within the room. As a consequence this results, in essence, in a mass healing taking place, everyone who is present within the room is involved to some extent. After Nicola had received her healing, and my consciousness returned to normal, I became aware that every member of the audience had a spirit healer who was standing behind them and was sending them healing energy. I then asked Nicola if she had felt, or experienced anything during the healing. She told me that she had experienced a feeling of tingling down the length of her body almost like pins and needles. In addition, Nicola stated that it felt as if someone had been working upon her kidneys.

After the demonstration I spoke to Nicola in order to find out a little more about her condition. She told me that had suffered from renal problems from birth and, over the years, had regularly attended hospital for investigations and treatment. Ten years ago, when she was thirty-two years old, her kidneys failed completely. She was commenced on renal dialysis and her husband underwent tests to see if he was compatible to donate a kidney. Fortunately this was the case and the transplant was performed in December 2005. Sadly the transplanted kidney threatened to reject almost immediately and she spent the next six years in and out of hospital trying to save it. However, eventually it failed completely and Nicola recommenced dialysis in February 2012.

Many family members and friends underwent tests to see if they were candidates to donate a kidney to Nicola but sadly none were compatible. Her specialist also advised Nicola that, even if a suitable kidney was to become available, owing to the problems that she had undergone during rejection of her husband's kidney, she now had raised levels of antibodies in her blood that would increase the risk of rejection. He explained that Nicola could face a long wait for a suitable donor organ and that the chance of her ever receiving a transplant was only around one percent. Obviously this was extremely upsetting to her. Life on dialysis is difficult.

Months passed and eventually Nicola contacted me through my website. She told me that she had been at a charity fundraising event for kidney research and that my friend, the medium who had shared the event with me during which I first met Jane, had been delivering a demonstration of mediumship. My friend, Jane Dawson, had strongly suggested that Nicola should book a series of four appointments with me at monthly intervals. She had also put her credibility on the line by telling Nicola that she felt that eventually a suitable kidney would be received from a male donor. Since Nicola was no longer on the transplant list this seemed to be unlikely.

Nicola said she that she felt that she had nothing to lose and told me that she had an open mind concerning spiritual healing.

The arrangements were made and the first of the healings took place a couple of weeks later at my Edinburgh clinic. As the healing energy began to blend with her energy Nicola would go to sleep. After each healing session she stated that she felt a lot better physically and that, in addition, she had a feeling of calmness that helped to make her more at ease with her situation.

The fourth healing session took place on October 2014. A week or so after the appointment, out of the blue, Nicola received a phone call from her consultant who told her that her antibodies had reduced to a level that she was now she was eligible for a transplant and her name had been added to the list. Since she had not been receiving any medical treatment that could have accounted this change in her levels of antibodies and the consultant was equally amazed as Nicola.

Nicola had one more appointment with me in November 2014 and I told her that I had a feeling that there was a good chance she would have a transplant before the end of the year. In December 2014 Nicola received a phone call to say that a kidney had become available for her. It turned out to be a perfect match and on the 14th of December 2014 Nicola underwent her surgery. Seven hours later she had her new kidney. The operation was a success. Everything went like clockwork; it was a textbook operation.

A few days later I received a call from my friend, the lady medium. She was a little concerned since Nicola had posted on Facebook that her kidney was not producing urine on its own accord. I told my friend not to worry and that everything would work out fine. I also sent Nicola a message, telling her I would link with my team later on that day and send distant healing to her.

I sat with my spirit team at 12.40 am and sent distant healing to Nicola. When the distant healing was taking place I was taken to her bedside at the hospital and had the privilege once again to work alongside my spirit team during the distant healing session. I watched as they put energy into her new kidney. I asked what the problem was with her kidney and was told that it just needed a 'kick-start' to get it going. I was with Nicola for about five to ten minutes, after which I was taken to visit some other people who were to receive distant healing.

The following morning Nicola announced on Facebook that her kidney had started to produce urine. This came as no surprise to me. I have since spoken to Nicola and have told her about visiting her through distant healing. In return she has informed me that, on the evening in question, a feeling of peacefulness had come over her and she knew that everything would be all right.

Nicola sent me a testimonial for my website and contained within it she has stated amongst other things, 'I cannot find the words to thank you both [Jane Dawson and me]. Jane, for urging me to see you; and you for the healing that I have received. Without it I honestly believe, I would not be here today.'

The most important thing in this whole process is the spirit intelligence behind the whole operation for it was them that organized for us all to meet that first time in Motherwell and when the time was right, for Nicola and Jane to meet up again at the charity fundraiser. As a consequence Nicola was able to connect with my spirit team and myself at the right time for everything to fall into place.

A Young Lady with a Brain Tumor

I have had the pleasure of getting to know a lovely young girl called Melissa and her mother, who came to visit me at my clinic in Johnstone. Melissa had undergone gone four operations to remove a tumor that was situated in the left side of her brain. After her mother had given me some background information concerning her daughter's health problem, we agreed to see what the Spirit World could do for her.

I was told that Melissa was attending high school and that,

owing to her condition, she would tire easily. As a consequence, each day she would require to take a nap for roughly an hour at a time in order conserve her energy sufficiently to get her through the day. Her mother told me that on several occasions she had taken Melissa to an alternative healing therapist but she felt that there had been no significant improvement in her daughter's general wellbeing. She proceeded to tell me that I had been recommended to her through a third party, which, to be honest, is how most of my clients learn of me ('the proof of the pudding is in the eating' as they say).

I asked Melissa to lie onto the massage table and to make herself as comfortable as she could. When the healing commenced she fell fast asleep and remained in that state for the duration of the healing session. This healing session was very emotional one for me. Never before had I felt such love and compassion from the Spirit side of life as I did on this occasion. I was aware that the people working through me were sending energy directly to that part of the young girl's head that was the site of the operation that had been undertaken to remove the tumor. I also became aware of my hands slowly waving around above the young girl's torso. They seemed to be playing in the energy that had been created around Melissa, in a controlled manner. It was as if the person working through me was like a conductor in charge of an orchestra. They were in perfect harmony with, and in complete control of, the healing energies. I could feel the love, not just from the spirit people, but also from Melissa's mother as she observed what was taking place.

The healing session lasted for about half an hour, following which the spirit people withdrew their energy from me. I particularly remember being very emotional, and I had a tear in my eye, when this healing session was finished. I looked at Melissa's mother and noted that she also had a tear in her eye.

I was quite astounded at what had taken place and knew that this manipulation of the energy in the air above the young girl was correct. I gently woke Melissa and arranged to see her again in a month's time. Since then, I have had the pleasure of working with Melissa several times. On each of these occasions her mother has informed me about the improvements that she has noticed in Melissa's health and general wellbeing. This young girl is a regular visitor to my clinic. She is turning into a lovely young lady and, from what I hear, is one to watch with the boys. Recently the mother received a letter from her Melissa's specialist and kindly forwarded the letter to me in order that it may be added to this story. The following is a direct extract from that letter:

We talked about Chris Ratter your Psychic Surgeon who certainly seems to have improved your mental state as well as your physical ability. This chap that you see in Edinburgh I believe, who sees you once a month, and I am not sure how he does it, but he promotes a sense of wellbeing and you have confidence in his ability. As a result you are walking better, you are not sleeping at school and are more active. This is all great news and long may it continue.

Thank you to Mellissa for allowing me to include this quote.

A Lady with No Sensations of Taste or Smell

Another case study that comes to mind involved a lady called Jackie. Jackie had lost her sense of smell and taste, and had been unable to pick up anything using these senses for a few months. I suppose we really never give a second thought to these senses that we have until they cease to function properly. It is only then that we become aware of how important they are to us our everyday lives. I had never heard of this condition before and was intrigued to see what the Spirit World could do to help.

Jackie lay on the massage table and closed her eyes and the connection was made with the Spirit World. Jackie's body started to react to the energy immediately and went into spasm. It jerked uncontrollably for a good few minutes before settling down once again. Sometimes this can happen when the healing energy connects with the energy of the person who is receiving the healing. Never be frightened if this should occur during the course of a healing. Trust in your spirit team at all times.

I was aware of healing energy in the form of colors that where flowing through my mind, these colors were travelling down through my body, out through my fingertips and into Jackie's head. I watched as the healing energy went up into the nasal passages, into the corners of her eyes and eventually into her mouth. At one stage the energy was present in all these places at the same time. I become aware of spirit instruments that were contained within these energies. These spirit instruments were being manipulated at an incredible speed around the area at which the energy was entering Jackie's face.

This continued for about five minutes, after which my guides caused me to sit down once again. After a few minutes they brought me back. Jackie had fallen asleep. When I woke her, she said that she had felt someone, or something, working at the back of her eyes. She reported that she had been aware also of things happening at the back of her nose and throat. 'That was WEIRD,' she said. (I find that this is a word that is used commonly by my clients to describe the feelings that they experience during a healing session.) I thanked her for the opportunity for allowing my spirit team to work with her and asked her to rest for twenty-four hours, to drink plenty of water and not to take any alcohol.

After she had left the room I could hear Jackie discussing what she had experienced with some other ladies in the waiting area. I overheard one of them saying, 'Wait a moment, I will light a vanilla incense stick and see if you can smell it.' I awaited the results of the experiment with some anticipation. What I heard next made me proud to be of service to Divine Spirit and to the people from the Spirit World. 'I CAN SMELL, I CAN SMELL,' I heard Jackie say from the next room.

Some Unusual Aspects
of Mediumship

One of my key purposes in writing this book is to share with my readers some of the wonderful things that I have experienced during my spiritual journey. Amazing though some of these may be, there have been others that, before I experienced them first-hand, I would have described as being both incredible and improbable. It would be remiss of me not to mention some of them here. The main message that I would ask you to take from them is to keep an open mind.

Strength in Mediumship

As mediums, we are expected to know everything about Spiritualism and how everything works concerning Spirit side of life. However, we are all constantly learning and sometimes we may feel insufficiently prepared to deal with issues that arise.

Throughout your spiritual journey there will be many difficult situations in which your help will be sought. There will come a time in your mediumship when your faith and knowledge will be tested. When situations arise with which you are unfamiliar, and you feel insufficiently experienced or prepared to address a particular issue, you should never consider it to be a failing to seek assistance from other experienced mediums.

Whenever we call upon them for help, the guides and helpers from the Spirit Realm who work with us will always assist, advise and protect us to the best of their ability. It is up to us to listen carefully to them, to ensure that we understand what they tell us, and to accept and follow whatever advice or information they give to us. It is important to be strong in your belief system at all times and to have strength in what you do for the Spirit World.

Astral Travel

I have had a few experiences of this phenomenon. The first one that I can recall was one evening when I was in an altered state of consciousness, and I became aware of a spirit guide who asked me to travel with him. I seemed to float out of my physical body, and travel with him to a world that was green in color.

We were floating above this strange world. Various gold symbols, contained within borders that looked like hedges, seemed to be strategically placed all over parts of the land. I could see sparkling lights in the distance, in the direction that we were travelling. When eventually we arrived at these sparkling lights, I realized that they were glass buildings that rose into a beautiful, blue skyline. There were quite a few of these buildings, all of which seemed to sparkle like sunlight, glistening on water. This place seemed to have a feeling of purity, peace and tranquility about it.

I was taken into one of these buildings through two glass doors that opened outwards, and entered a large area where many people were sitting or standing, having conversations with each other. None one seemed to have any cares. Everyone seemed to have all the time in the world. They were oblivious to us, as we seemed to float above them. I asked the spirit guide what I was seeing. 'This is a level where people come who do not wish to accept that they have passed over from your world,' he replied. 'These people do not wish to have change in their lives at this time. They are not spiritually ready to advance yet.'

We proceeded to travel across to the far end of the large room, towards what appeared to look like a glass lift. When we arrived at the lift the floating sensation stopped, and we found ourselves standing in front of the lift doors. I found myself looking at the glass around the lift area. It seemed to extend upward forever into the sky. After a few moments the lift door opened, and we both entered. Instantly the doors closed behind us, and we began to ascend.

The doors opened when we reached the next level, and we stepped out into a glass foyer. A beautiful lady who was sitting at a glass desk greeted us. Her energy was wonderful and she spoke so softly. 'Welcome, welcome,' she said. 'You can proceed no further at this time.' Then, all of a sudden, a beautiful bright white light appeared and started to expand outwards above her head. We turned round and proceeded to re-enter the lift. Once again, immediately we entered the lift the glass doors closed behind us. When they reopened, I was aware that I was back in my bedroom. I then knew that this was Spirit's way of showing me there are many levels of spiritual planes of existence.

Another experience that I had concerning astral travel occurred once again when I was at home, in bed. I awoke from sleep at 11.10am, after being visited by my father's spirit that had astral travelled to visit me. He had been suffering, both mentally and physically, from prostate gland problems for quite some time. When I was asleep I had become aware of my father sitting at the foot of my bed.

I remember speaking to him and asking him why he was there. He said that he had come to my house to have a rest from the suffering, associated with his condition. I recall telling him, 'Your spirit is strong.' He just sat there on the end of my bed for a few more moments and then disappeared, after which I woke up. I pondered over this experience for a few minutes, thinking to myself about the events that had just taken place. Then I went back to sleep.

I phoned my father later that day. I know you will be wondering why did I not phone right away but I knew he was all right, I just knew. Anyway, when I spoke to him and asked what he had been doing at approximately eleven o'clock that morning, he replied that he was meditating, and had become aware of a white light that had surrounded his head. This was a strange experience for me since he had astral travelled to me, and although I was aware of him having done so, he was not.

Everyone's experiences of astral travel are unique. Our guides know exactly how our minds work. If you allow your mind to be open to them, who knows where they could take you, what wonders you will experience, and how this will further your understanding.

House Clearing

House clearing is a specific form of mediumship in which the medium acts as an intermediary to enable spirit guides to move earth-bound and visiting spirits into the light if required. This is not something that should be taken lightly. There may be personal risks to the medium. In addition, there is the potential to exacerbate the situation that it is desired to resolve. Those who undertake this role require to be experienced mediums who have strength and confidence in their mediumship. They must also have complete trust in their spirit workers.

My first experience of assisting an earth-bound spirit to move into the light

I was asked to help a family that were experiencing strange phenomena in their home. Within their home, vases were being turned round and other objects were being moved around. Their dog would bark constantly at the living room door. Their twin daughters would wake up screaming in the middle of the night, and would speak of seeing a lady with one arm standing in the corner of their bedroom. Photographs that had been taken of the young children showed a large amount of 'orb' activity.

I had only been in a development class for mental mediumship for six to eight months and, although I felt quite confident in my mediumship, I had the common sense to ask an experienced medium to accompany me to investigate these strange events. We arrived at their home at two o'clock in the afternoon. We were invited in, taken into the sitting room, and offered a cup of tea. The lady went into the kitchen. Meanwhile her husband, and the experienced medium (whom I shall call Margaret) and I sat together in the sitting room.

After a few minutes had passed, Margaret turned to me and asked if I was experiencing anything. I told her that I was aware of a gentleman from Spirit who was standing at the door observing us. 'Very good,' she said, and then proceeded to give the householder a reading from his parents in Spirit. When this was finished she turned to me once again and asked, 'Is he still standing at the door?'

'Yes,' I replied.

'Ask him to come forward and speak to you,' she said. I did as I was instructed and could feel the spirit gentleman's energy starting to draw closer to me. Margaret instructed me to ask him why he was there and I sent the thought to him.

'I live here. This is my home and my family,' he replied. I asked him if he had been responsible for turning the vase around. 'Yes, it is my vase and it keeps getting turned the wrong way round,' was his reply.

It transpired that the gentleman's wife had passed over a number of years before him. He told me that she had suffered a stroke that had rendered her left arm limp. When the gentleman passed over a few years later he had somehow made himself earth-bound and still considered this to be his own home. When the new family moved in, he had attached himself to the children. His wife would often return from the light and would attempt to contact him as he stood watch over the children. Although the children were aware of the lady, they could not see the gentleman.

Next Margaret asked me to tell the gentleman that we were we are going to 'put him to the light'. As soon as I said this I felt the gentleman's energy rapidly leave the room. Margaret told me to follow him. As I went into the hall I was aware of a green mass of light over the children's bedroom door.

'He is in there,' I said.

'Well go on in,' was her reply.

Into the bedroom we went and closed the door behind us. We could feel his energy standing in front of us, in the middle of the room. 'We know you are a little confused,' said Margaret, 'but we are going to help you to cross over to the light.' I started to speak to the gentleman asking him if he was aware of the light and telling him to go into the light. Then all of a sudden we could feel his energy running around us. When I say running around us, I mean we could feel his energy moving around us very quickly as if he was in a panic. He was trying to hide from us and to stay away from the light. Eventually the gentleman's energy began to settle and he started to listen to what was being said to him. After a few minutes we were aware of him heading towards the light and taking the hand of his wife. He had crossed over.

During the events that had just taken place, it had been very cold in the room and the temperature now returned to normal. What an experience, but fortunately it had been performed under the supervision and guidance of a medium who was experienced in dealing with this sort of problem.

Ghost in the House

I was asked by a lady to help with a ghost in her house; the lady had contacted me out of concern for her daughter. The young girl was seeing people standing in her bedroom in the middle of the night and was too scared to stay in her own room. The mother and a friend were also experiencing inexplicable strong putrid smells around the house. I agreed to see if I could help, and arranged a time to visit the house. A few days later, my wife and I arrived at a Georgian terraced house in Edinburgh. The lady invited us in and offered to make us coffee. As I sat drinking my coffee I became aware of a male figure that was standing at the top of the stairs.

I asked the lady if it was all right for me to have a look around her home. The house had three storeys. The child's bedroom was on the first level. It was here that the gentleman from Spirit had been standing when I first noticed him. I went into the room and sat on the child's bed for a short while. I then became aware of the presence of a spirit lady who was standing at the entrance to the child's bedroom. I acknowledged her presence and said, 'Hello.'

The lady explained that she was trying to help the little girl and to comfort her.

I then became aware of the presence of the gentleman once again. He was standing in the hallway. I told him that his presence was scaring the little girl.

'This is my home,' he replied.

'Not anymore, your time has passed,' I told him. 'You may still visit here from time to time, but these people live here now.'

At this I felt the gentleman getting angry. I remember thinking to myself, 'You need to go to the light.' As quick as a flash, he said, 'You are not strong enough to put me to the light.'

I must admit, that did catch me off guard, and for a split second, I doubted myself. Then I regained my composure. 'Oh yes I am,' was my reply.

Now, although these conversations take place in thought form, nonetheless they are real. In this kind of situation, I always ask Divine Spirit and my spirit team to assist and to protect me. The battle of minds went on for quite some time until eventually my spirit protectors, through their love and compassion, assisted the gentleman to walk into the light.

The lady has had no further visits from this gentleman from Spirit. I thank the Divine Spirit and his helpers for what they did. This spirit gentleman was testing the strength of my faith in my belief in the Divine Spirit and my spirit team. This was the second time I had been involved in a house clearing. Since then there have been several more, but it is the one that I will relate to you next, that really tested my strength as a medium.

A Scary Encounter

I was invited to visit commercial premises in Edinburgh, the owner of which was worried that it might be haunted. Having recently acquired the building, they were concerned about a series of inexplicable happenings. Formerly a launderette, it had been fully refurbished and converted into a fabulous restaurant. From the start, it had been plagued with electrical surges. The premises had been completely rewired from top to bottom, but still brand new appliances would stop working for no apparent reason. They consulted electrician after electrician who carried out extensive testing, both of the wiring circuits and of the appliances, all to no avail. For the owner, the last straw happened one Saturday night shortly after the restaurant had opened.

It was full of customers and everything was in full swing. Suddenly the toilet door flew open and a customer came running out shouting that a ghost had appeared in front of him when he was in the toilet. To everyone's consternation and horror, he had been in such a fluster that he had fled the toilet without taking the time to pull up his trousers.

Together with another developing medium, my wife and nephew, I went to visit the restaurant one Sunday afternoon when it was closed to the public. Standing outside the restaurant as we waited for the owner to arrive, I could sense a heavy dense energy associated with the premises. It felt horrible, oppressive, and full of negativity.

The lady arrived and after exchanging pleasantries, we entered the building. We sat down and over a coffee the lady described the events that had been taking place, along with her concerns. While we were sitting chatting, I was aware of a spirit lady at the far end of the room who just ignored us and went about her business. I was also very much aware that the focus of the oppressive energy was in the basement.

We went down the stairs to the basement, and the energy grew stronger. It seemed to affect my stomach; I started to feel nauseous. The basement was not what I was expecting. It was a lovely cellar bar, fresh looking, old with a touch of modern, but the spirit energy was heavy.

People don't mean to stir up spirit energy, but it often happens when they start to make alterations to old properties or to change the décor. If spirit people are attached to the building they may dislike what is happening to their former home. This was the situation in this restaurant. The new owner had opened-up and completely restructured the cellar in order to develop the business.

In the cellar, I sat on an armchair and asked Gail and the developing medium to sit opposite me so that we could all experience the feel of the energy in the cellar. After a short period of time had elapsed, I felt myself entering into an altered state of trance. When the blending process had taken place a gentleman came forward and asked me to request the proprietor to come forward and to sit opposite me.

The lady who owned the restaurant swapped places with my wife and sat opposite me, alongside the developing medium. Gail went back up the stairs. The gentleman spoke about his displeasure at what they had done to the premises. He explained that he had been there before them, and that he was not going anywhere in the near future. 'These premises are used by us,' he said. 'We have gathered here for a long time. There are portals in the cellar that we use for travel.' He proceeded to tell us that he had been responsible for some, but not all, of the untoward events that had happened since she had made the changes to the building.

The lady apologized to the spirit gentleman and explained that she meant no harm. She asked if there was anything she could do to appease the situation. 'Just acknowledge that we are here,' he said. 'Allow us to come and go as we please, and we will cease interfering in your business.'

The lady agreed and I returned from the altered state of

trance. My friend, the developing medium, said that the person who had come through gave her an eerie feeling. His head had been shrouded in a hood and he brought with him a black energy that surrounded his head, chest and face. When we went home, we decided to search the Internet for information about the area in which the restaurant was situated. To our surprise it is directly in the center of the place where the witches were held in Edinburgh before being sent for trial. The whole area is synonymous with occult and witchcraft.

What happened next tested my trust, faith and strength of my belief in my mediumship. I was lying in bed, when I became aware of the gentleman from Spirit that I had contacted in the basement of the restaurant, standing at the bottom of my bed. He did not say anything; he just stood there.

It was an extremely unsettling experience. I told him to leave but he did not. He just stood there, I asked my guides to intervene and to take him away. He went, only to re-appear. This went on for days and nights, I could not tell Gail; I did not want to alarm her. I trusted my spirit protectors and I knew that I was strong enough to show this spirit gentleman that there was no way he was going to attach himself to me. Eventually his visits ceased.

Some mischievous spirits will attach themselves to people whose minds are easily influenced. You must be strong if you want to engage with spirit entities, especially if you want to be involved in house clearings. Although I find this branch of mediumship to be fascinating, it is something I would not like to do every day. Nevertheless it is worth being aware that this is an aspect of mediumship in which some choose to specialize and that has an important function.

People must be careful when engaging with the Spirit Realm; there are many things that we do not understand. Although we can become aware of spirit people, not all of them want to engage with us; sometimes it is better to let sleeping dogs lie.

Elementals

I believe there are many strange, wonderful life forms in our world that we know little about. Who knows what we might become aware of, if we are lucky enough to be in the right place at the right time? Over the years I have read many books on the subject of mediumship. In some of them, reference is made to strange elemental beings that have been encountered during séances. We are unaware of what purpose these strange creatures serve in our world or from where they come.

My First Encounter with an Elemental

My first experience of these elementals occurred when I was sitting in an open circle in Edinburgh. I had been attending this awareness group for several months. It was a lovely group, comprising people with various levels of mediumistic development. After sitting in meditation for approximately half an hour, I had an uncontrollable desire to open my eyes. As I did so, my attention was drawn to a small table that was situated in the center of the group, and was directly in front of me. I blinked my eyes.

I could not believe what I was seeing. A little green fairy lady, roughly twelve inches in height, was looking back at me. She was absolutely beautiful and delicate. She sat on the edge of the table in front of me, swinging her legs backwards and forwards. After about five seconds she disappeared. I couldn't believe what I had just seen. I shared my experience with the group, and waited to be ridiculed by them. The circle leader said that another gentleman who had attended their group some years previously, reported seeing fairies on the very same table. Strangely enough, these were also green.

When sitting in awareness groups or development circles, it is important that you recount anything that you see, hear or feel. If, on this occasion, had I failed to do so, I would not have received confirmation that these lovely little fairy people had been seen previously in the very same room. I was also told by the circle leader that green is the most common color for fairies. We don't really understand why these elemental beings show themselves to us. One thing that we do know is that, in order for us to become aware of them, we have to be in tune with their energies.

A Tree Spirit Appears During Our Trance Development Group

I was sitting one night in my home for physical trance development. There were four of us in the development circle that evening. One of the regular sitters was a gentleman who is a wonderfully talented artist. We were sitting observing some spirit helpers, working with energy around the head of a lady, who was sitting in the séance cabinet under red light conditions. A séance cabinet is covered on the roof and on three sides with material drapes. There are also drapes at the front that may either be left open or closed as required. This type of cabinet is used to harness trance energy, for development purposes.

All of a sudden we were aware that the energy within the séance room had changed. Unusually, it had become very hot. Normally it is very cold in a séance room when a séance, or development is taking place. The energy within the room seemed to come alive. It felt as though the room had become charged with electricity.

This was an energy that I had never experienced previously in any séance room. I became aware then of the presence of energy to my right, and focused my attention upon it. As I did so, I became conscious of a small figure, approximately two feet tall, which was standing in the séance room, next to the door to my kitchen. It appeared to be in the form of a tiny man, with skin that looked like the bark of a tree.

'What is this that has joined our development circle?' I

thought. I could not take my eyes off this strange, little creature. It did not speak. It just stood there motionless. Whatever it was, it seemed to have brought with it this beautiful strange, hot energy, which had electrified the room. I asked the other sitters if any of them were aware of anything unusual in the room. The gentleman in our group who is a very talented artist confirmed that he was aware of this little chap, and was excited that he was not the only one to see him.

I asked my spirit guide to explain to me what we were witnessing. He replied that it was an elemental: a tree spirit, that had visited the circle. He explained that they bring an energy that is required for physical mediumship, and it is very rare for them to show themselves. This little man stayed for about ten minutes, after which he disappeared as suddenly as he had arrived.

A few weeks later, the artist gentleman who had also witnessed this event, presented me with the most beautiful drawing of the strange little tree spirit who had blessed us with his presence that evening. This picture has a special place on my wall in my home. I did not know what a tree spirit was until he had graced us with his presence that evening. Since the events that took place that evening, I have done a little research into what they are and I have found out that tree spirits are involved with healing, which ties nicely in with my own journey.

A Blending of Energies

Sometimes the Spirit World will put a thought into your mind and it will not go away. One day I felt compelled to go for a walk, and to become immersed in the freedom of nature. It was a sunny, Sunday afternoon, so Gail and I we went out for a drive. We ended up at a place that is very dear to my heart, the village of Blackness. This village has a 15th-century fortress nearby called Blackness Castle. The castle has lots of history attached to it. In the mid 1400s it served as a state prison. In 1650 it was besieged and taken by the army of Oliver Cromwell. The army also used it during World War One.

I have previously mentioned that I had spent a lot of my childhood at this location as my grandfather and granny lived there for many years. My grandfather worked for Historic Scotland and was the castle custodian there for many years before his retirement. I still go back there from time-to-time to walk in the grounds.

Gail and I took a slow walk along the shoreline and headed towards the wooded area of Blackness. Just before we entered the woods I felt drawn to sit down at a grassy area alongside a small stream. After a few minutes of sitting there relaxing, and becoming one with the energy around me, I decided to meditate.

Shortly after starting my meditation I became aware of a spirit guide, who started to speak to me. He informed me that there were elementals that wished to join me, and to attune themselves to my energies. I was intrigued by this, and excited by the events that I was about to experience.

After a few moments I became aware of circles of light drawing close and forming a circle around me. I was very aware that these elemental beings were all different in size and form, and that the light energies they brought with them varied, both in intensity and size. Their energies began to blend with my own, forming one mass of white light. I was then entertained with the most beautiful colors, some of which I had never seen before. This blending of their energy with mine was harmonizing. For a short time it made me feel one with my surroundings and with them.

This wonderful experience continued for approximately half an hour. After this, all of a sudden, the energy that we had become encased in rose upwards in a spiral motion and dissipated. No verbal communication took place between us as we blended and sat in the energy, there was no need. I came away from this experience with the understanding that we are all one with the planet.

In the busy world in which we live, we have become unaware of these things. It is a great privilege when we are invited to link with beings such as these, as I was. Moments like this will never be forgotten. They will be cherished forever. Although these strange, but incredible, life forms are all around us, to many they seem fanciful. I am aware that elemental beings are involved in healing and physical mediumship.

Some Funny Stories

There is nothing stranger than working with the public, here are some events in my healing journey that made me chuckle. I have not used anyone's names as I do not wish to cause any embarrassment to them.

A Strange Gift from a Client

I was working in my Edinburgh clinic, and my next appointment was running late. When the doorbell rang I opened the door, and two ladies, a mother and her daughter, confronted me. They had been having problems with the satellite navigation in the car and had been unable to find the clinic. Consequently they were flustered and anxious about being late for the appointment. After the introductions were made, the older of the two ladies (the mother) said, 'This is for you,' and handed me a blue carrier bag.

Oh, I thought, *how lovely she has given me a present. I hope it's scones.* 'That's lovely,' I said. 'Thank you, what is it?'

'Oh that's a bag of sick,' she replied. 'I didn't know what to do with it.'

'That's nice,' I thought to myself as I took it outside to deposit it in the bucket!

An Elongated Story

On another occasion I was holding a healing clinic in Glasgow. A lovely lady that I had worked with previously had returned for a follow up appointment. The lady was speaking to my wife Gail. They had been talking for a few minutes before I was invited into the conversation. The lady said that when she was here last time at the clinic, I had worked upon her elongated testicles (she meant twisted intestines). 'I can't remember working on them,' was my reply! Once the lady had realized what she had said, she was mortified. When she saw Gail doubled over with laughter, she too had a fit of the giggles. There is something good contained in the power of laughter.

Pillow Talk

Another quick one that comes to mind is when for the first time I had spoken to a lady regarding her condition, I asked her to please get on to the massage table. She asked at which end would I like her head? So I said, 'Please put your head on the pillow.'

The lady proceeded to put her head on the pillow without getting on the bed, and stood there bent over for quite some time. Like an emu sticking its head into the sand, I looked over at the lady's daughter, who just burst out laughing! Needless to say, as soon as the lady realized the error of her ways she then lay correctly on the bed.

Reflections

Mine has been a personal journey of discovery. In this book I have attempted to encapsulate key aspects of my development to date. It has been an exciting journey and no one (on the material plane) knows where it will lead me in the future. My purpose in writing this book is twofold. Firstly, for those who decide to pursue actively their involvement with Spirit, to provide them with some reference points.

We all have doubts from time-to-time. It is easy to attempt to judge our progress against that of others, to covet their gifts and to feel inferior to them. No two journeys are the same. No one is better, more powerful, or more important than anyone else. Each of us is unique. We all have our own special gifts. It is up to us to recognize what these are and to use them for the greatest possible benefit for all (not only for individuals or even for mankind but for all things in this universe and beyond).

As we work with the gifts that we have, the Spirit World will offer us opportunities to develop them and to acquire others. Nonetheless when you are experiencing the 'ups and downs' and are questioning yourself, your own abilities and the existence of Spirit, it is useful to see that it is not just you that have these doubts. It is a function of mediumship.

By recounting aspects of my development I hope that I have been able to show that when you learn to trust yourself and more importantly, those who choose to come forward from the Spirit World to work with and through you, many things are possible. Remember this – for in my experience it has always been the case – as one doors closes, another opens. It is up to you whether you wish to step through. We all have free will.

My second purpose is to provide with you with some practical guidance: some pointers about how to progress some aspects of mediumship that are based upon my own experience.

During my journey I have met, worked with, and have received teaching and guidance from a great many wonderful people. Nonetheless there have been times during my development when I have encountered new things and have been unable to find anyone with the particular skills and experience to help me to make sense of what was happening. In some cases there have been events and issues in relation to which I was unable to find anything in published material, either in books, journal articles or even on the Internet.

When this has been the case I have sought guidance from my friends, both in the Spirit World and in this, the material world. Together we have experimented, and have arrived at answers and methods that we have found helpful to us, and that has enabled us to move forward. For your information I have attempted to include some of these in this book. However, it was never my intention to provide a practical guide to mediumship or mediumship by numbers. In my experience there is no single formula that applies to all. What works for one may not work for another. For example, practical visualization techniques are of no value (and indeed could be a turn-off) for those of you who are unable to visualize.

Much has been published about how to develop as a medium. I can see how it might be easy to follow the teachings of a particular person (a role model or someone that is, or has been widely admired) and to limit oneself to particular techniques or methods that may have been appropriate to them. There may be many ways of achieving the same outcome. My advice is to keep an open mind, listen to all that others have to say, read widely, experiment and listen to your higher self, your spirit guides and friends. Try not to become bound by ritual. It is not necessary and once it becomes ingrained, it may stifle your progress.

Let me emphasize a few simple points of guidance that, if followed will keep support your development and keep you safe as you progress along your spiritual path. Firstly, I would wish to emphasize the importance of development groups and circles as a means of progressing your development, particularly, but not exclusively, during the early stages of your development. There is nothing better, or more comforting than developing together with, and under the guidance of others. Many of those people that you meet in this way will become long-term friends, guides and teachers.

Avoid ego. This is abhorrent to the Spirit World. As I have said, no one is person better than the next. Those who consider themselves to be a 'cut above' the rest are setting themselves up for a fall. Use your gifts for the greatest benefit of all. Do not be tempted to seek to use them for any form of personal gain. This is a dangerous route and must be avoided. Linked with this, do not envy others their gifts. This will only serve to block your own development.

Finally, keep yourself safe. Heed the advice of those who have more experience than you in a particular aspect of mediumship. Ask for protection before working with Spirit and avoid situations in which you feel exposed. Listen to your spirit guides. Remember to seek their guidance, protection and help at all times.

By reading this book you have demonstrated your interest in developing along your spiritual path. Many of you will already have made considerable progress. I have no doubt that, as long as you follow these few simple suggestions and advice, this will be a wonderful journey for you.

Reference

1. Ramus Branch, 1982. *Harry Edwards: The life story of the great healer*. Tiptree, Essex, The Anchor Press Ltd.

BOOKS

6th Books investigates the paranormal, supernatural, explainable or unexplainable. Titles cover everything included within parapsychology: how to, lifestyles, beliefs, myths, theories and memoir.

www.6th-books.com

If this book has helped you to clarify an idea, solve a problem or extend your knowledge,
you may like to read other 6th-Books titles on parapsychology. Recent bestsellers are:

The Afterlife Unveiled
What the dead are telling us about their world
Stafford Betty
What happens after we die? Spirits speaking through mediums know. They want us to know. This book unveils their world.
Paperback: 2011, 978-1-84694-496-3 $16.95 £9.99
eBook: 978-1-84694-926-5 $9.99 £6.99

Less Incomplete
A Guide to Experiencing the Human Condition beyond the Physical Body
Sandie Gustus
Based on 40 years of scientific research, this book is a dynamic guide to understanding life beyond the physical body.
Paperback: 2011, 978-1-84694-351-5 $26.95 £15.99
eBook: 978-1-84694-892-3 $9.99 £6.99

I'm Still With You
True Stories of Healing Grief Through Spirit Communication
Carole J. Obley
These stories uplift, comfort and heal and show how love helps us grieve.
Paperback: 2008, 978-1-84694-107-8 $22.95 £11.99
eBook: 978-1-84694-639-4 $9.99 £6.99

Spirit Release
Sue Allen
A guide to psychic attack, curses, witchcraft, spirit attachment, possession, soul retrieval, haunting, soul rescue, deliverance, exorcism and others as taught at the College of Psychic Studies in London.
Paperback: 2007, 978-1-84694-033-0 $24.95 £11.99
eBook: 978-1-84694-651-6 $9.99 £6.99

Advanced Psychic Development
Becky Walsh
Learn how to practise as a professional contemporary spiritual medium
Paperback: 2007, 978-1-84694-062-0 $22.95 £9.99
eBook: 2012, 978-1-78099-941-8 $9.99 £6.99.

Audible Life Stream
The Ancient Secret of Dying While Living
Alistair Conwell
The secret to unlocking your purpose in life is solving the mystery of death while still living.
Paperback: 2010, 978-1-84694-329-4 $24.95 £11.99.

Divine Guidance
The answers you need to make miracles
Stephanie J. King
Ask a question – any question – and the answer will immediately be presented, like a direct line – a telephone link – to the higher realms...
Paperback: 2013, 978-1-78099-794-0 $11.95 £7.99
eBook: 2013, 978-1-78099-793-3 $9.99 £6.99.

The End of Death
How Near-Death Experiences Prove the Afterlife
Admir Serrano
A compelling examination of Near Death Experience, proving immortality in every page.
Paperback: 2013, 978-1-78279-233-8 $19.95 £11.99
eBook: 2013, 978-1-78279-232-1 $9.99 £6.99

Miracle Workers Handbook
The Seven Levels of Power and Manifestation of the Virgin Mary
Sherrie Dillard
Teaches how to invoke the Virgin Marys presence, communicate with her, receive her grace and miracles and become a miracle worker.
Paperback: 2012, 978-1-84694-920-3 $22.95 £12.99
eBook: 2012, 978-1-84694-921-0 $9.99 £6.99

Soul to Soul Connections
Comforting Messages from the Spirit World
Carole J. Obley
How to heal relationships with deceased loved ones and open our hearts to grow spiritually.
Paperback: 2012 978-1-84694-967-8 $22.95 £12.99
eBook: 2012 978-1-84694-968-5 $9.99 £6.99

Astral Projection Made Easy
Overcoming the fear of death
Stephanie Sorrell
Man's greatest fear is the fear of death, this book helps to eliminate this fear.
Paperback: 2012 978-1-84694-611-0 $9.95 £4.99
eBook: 2012 978-1-78099-225-9 $3.99 £2.99

Electronic Voices: Contact with Another Dimension?
Anabela Cardoso
Career diplomat and experimenter Dr Anabela Cardoso covers
the latest research into instrumental transcommunication ITC
and electronic voice phenomena EVP.
Paperback: 2010, 978-1-84694-363-8 $24.95 £14.99

Multidimensional Evolution
Personal Explorations of Consciousness
Kim McCaul
Once you understand your multidimensional nature, you can
make every moment count.
Paperback: 2013 978-1-78279-088-4 $22.95 £12.99
eBook: 2013 978-1-78279-089-1 $7.99 £4.99